TYPE 2 DIABETES NAVIGATION GUIDE

FOR EVERYONE OF AFRICAN, MIDDLE EASTERN, AND SOUTH ASIAN DESCENT

This book is being given to

_____

because I care about you, your health, and well-being.

_____

Comments from beta readers
of
Type 2 Diabetes Navigation Guide

"As a General Practitioner with a special interest in diabetes, I feel there is a need for clear and jargon-free evidence-based information that can be provided for patients with type 2 diabetes. This book fills that gap, and the format is easy to follow."

Dr. Paula Fernandes (Diabetes GPwSI Lead NHS North West London ICB)

"An excellent, informative, and easily digestible book which will help many people living with diabetes take control of their destiny. A must read!"

Dr. Noorez Hirani (Diabetes GPwSI Lead NHS Hammersmith & Fulham Partnership PCN)

"This is a very well written teaching tool for diabetes management for the general public and for clinicians. Thanks for simplifying the content without compromising the information. Both clinician and patient will enjoy informative review consultation sessions. The myths about the condition, diet, medication, natural herbs have been well addressed. A really simple and practical navigation!"

Sibongile Thembi Xaba (Practice Diabetes Nurse, NHS North West London)

"This book helps to educate you about Type 2 diabetes – and empowers you to do something about it. It explains how you can reverse or manage your diabetes providing a step-by-step plan which includes ethnically diverse foods from around the world highlighting how to make diet and lifestyle changes that can be sustained."
Dr Adel Isaak (GPwSI in Diabetes, NHS Hammersmith & Fulham Centres for Health)

"With this book Tembi is sharing what she's learned from thousands of consultations. In doing so she's created a guide that is as useful for professionals as it is for those living with diabetes. The content is comprehensive, practical, and focused not only on giving information, but on generating understanding so people can apply this to their own contexts. The chapters are engaging, enjoyable and make complex concepts easy to understand. It's a fantastic book and I'll be recommending this to patients and colleagues alike."
Dr Chad Hockey (GP and North PCN Clinical Director NHS Hammersmith & Fulham)

"This book is truly transformative! It's like a personalized guide for people from diverse ethnic backgrounds, helping them navigate their health journey easily. The content is not only easy to understand but also interesting, making it accessible to everyone. Whether you're curious about staying healthy, trying to prevent diabetes, or managing the condition, this book has answers for you.
It covers a range of topics, offering insights into healthy habits, preventing diabetes, and making lifestyle changes. It's a valuable resource for anyone looking for guidance on wellness, diabetes prevention, or effective management. This book is more than just reading; it's a powerful tool that empowers and enlightens. A must-read for all!"
Chakshu Sharma (An appreciative reader of Indian descent and Manager in the NHS North West London ICB)

TYPE 2 DIABETES NAVIGATION GUIDE

FOR EVERYONE OF AFRICAN, MIDDLE EASTERN, AND SOUTH ASIAN DESCENT

Tembi Chinaire

Diabetes Educator, Certified Nutrition Adviser
and
Diabetes Consultant Nurse

Pepukai Press
London, United Kingdom

A CIP catalogue record of this book is available
from the British Library.

ISBN-Print 978-1-9161967-2-8 |E-book 978-1-9161967-3-5
Printed by Ingram Spark

Design & Layout © Kiri Chinaire
Cover & Images © Saba Shafiq

Disclaimer: Information in this book is for general pur-
poses only and should not be considered as a substitute
for medical expertise.
The publisher and the author are not responsible for any
specific health needs that may require medical supervision.
The reader should seek professional help regarding any
health conditions and concerns.

This book is dedicated to countless patients who put into practice what they learned and became drivers of their own healthcare.

Contents

CHAPTER 1

Introduction

If I wasn't a diabetes healthcare professional and had never lost family members to the disease I would probably have no incentive to know more about type 2 diabetes. But I am in the same boat as millions of people of African, South Asian, or Middle Eastern descent who know at least four or five people who have been diagnosed with type 2 diabetes, pre-diabetes, or diabetes in pregnancy and have seen the effects of diabetes-related complications.

Why a book about people of African, South Asian, and Middle Eastern descent? The common ground includes a high incidence of diagnosis of type 2 diabetes and the prevalence of diabetes-related complications. Statistics published by the World Health Organization (WHO) and the International Diabetes Federation (IDF) confirm the reality that diabetes-related deaths continue to rise.

Countless families are living with daily reminders of the recurring devastation to normal life caused by type 2 diabetes. Poor healthcare services in some regions and health inequalities compound the epidemic and impede proactivity. Consequently, a significant percentage of adults living with diabetes are undiagnosed.

Fact-based formal diabetes education competes with half-truths, myths, cultural and religious beliefs, and claims of little-known instant remedies. An abundance of information in the public domain has not yet translated into knowledge for those who need it the most; there is a general lack of knowledge of what needs to be known about the disease.

Some find comfort in this lack of knowledge and proclaim, "What I don't know won't hurt me." But the reality is that the less you know about type 2 diabetes, the more vulnerable you are. This book answers some of the questions you may have and promotes self-care to prevent, reverse, or manage diabetes. Self-care is the new currency in today's health economy.

CHAPTER 2

Exploring Reasons for the Rise

This chapter explores some of the drivers, cultural norms, and societal values that make people of African, Middle Eastern, and South Asian descent fertile ground for type 2 diabetes. Understanding what is hardwired in the subconscious may provide pointers to what needs to be unlearned.

Belief that diabetes is inevitable

Many sincerely believe diabetes is inevitable because of their family's history of the disease. Unlike HIV infection which had a stigma, diabetes is readily accepted in the community, and the growing "diabetes club" is more welcoming.

Countless have subconsciously resigned themselves to developing and living with type 2 diabetes at "some" stage in their lives.

Carbohydrates are safe ground

Most food-related taboos, religious or cultural pertain to meats (proteins). The list includes cows are holy; pigs are unclean; and meat from animals linked to one's totem, heritage, or ancestry is prohibited.

Carbohydrates are generally considered safe and make up most of the food prepared at home and religious and cultural gatherings. They are, therefore, consumed in large quantities.

Propensity to overeat

Extended-family gatherings, cultural get-togethers, religious festivals, and celebrations provide ready excuses to overeat. In parts of Africa and the Middle East food is dished out and eaten communally, making it difficult to gauge how much one has consumed.

In homes, preparing and giving food to guests is an expression of love. Visiting family and friends one after another, particularly after a lengthy absence, carries the risk of reversing every discipline put into place. Most of the foods prepared are high in carbohydrates, and it is considered impolite to eat small amounts.

Fast foods, refined grains, and high-sugar foods

The increase in fast-food outlets everywhere and the promotion of refined grains have altered eating habits in Africa, the Middle East, and South Asia.

The first marketing campaigns for processed and refined foods were so effective that they defined food shopping and wish lists decades ahead of time. Super-refined grain products are desired more than whole grain, and many perceive processed foods as the epitome of good living.

Despite efforts by national advertising standards bodies, foods high in sugar, salt, and processed fat are still being promoted in many regions. The consequences will be felt for a long time. For example, a bodybuilder named "Powerman" promoted Goldstar white sugar in the 1970s in Rhodesia (now Zimbabwe). The superhero handed out cubes of sugar to school children, promising them they would be as strong as he was.

Despite the evidence of the negative impact of too much sugar on human health, the demand for white sugar is still high in most of sub-Saharan Africa and the West Indies.

Survival mode

Natural and man-made disasters of the past, such as wars, famines, slavery, colonisation, and political instability, pushed people into survival mode and made the victims choiceless. People ate what they were given or what was available, and this dictated their lifestyle.

The same is true today for people on the wrong end of forced migration, poverty, political instability, and recessions. Healthcare tends to take a back seat when survival is the driver. Prolonged survival mode passes "new norms" between generations, including unhealthy eating habits.

Personal healthcare is not a priority

Education and making a living are often prioritised above personal health. Education has long been seen as a ticket out of poverty for Africans and Asians across the globe.

Parents with little or no education don't need persuasion to appreciate the value of their children's education.

Healthcare only comes into play in times of illness. And even then, the focus is on quick fixes from any recommended source. The latest community health fads are often tried out before consulting healthcare professionals. For example, countless in parts of Southern Africa consumed quail eggs after being led to believe they were a "cure" for diabetes without making any lifestyle changes.

There is generally little appreciation or incentive to gather diabetes knowledge, make changes, and pass the information on to family members.

Outsourcing of personal healthcare

Only a minority assumes responsibility for their healthcare. The majority outsources it to healthcare professionals, spiritual healers, the church/temple, or a combination of the three. Diabetes is seen as a medical condition that is managed outside of the home and by the individual. The path that points to healing without making any changes to diet or lifestyle has the largest following.

Reduction of physical activity

All age groups have become less active over time. Progression has taken away incidental activities like walking, manual work, etc. Extreme heat conditions in the Middle East make it difficult to undertake most incidental activities. Some cities in developed countries have no sidewalks, forcing people to drive everywhere.

Driving to work is a status symbol, a step up the social ladder in many communities in Africa and South Asia. Public transport, cycling, or walking to work is for people lower down the social ladder. The affluent are often waited on hand and foot and do minimal activities. Manual work is left to hired hands and the poor.

Conscious effort and planning are now needed to do the minimum, like walking. On the other hand, the amount of food consumed has either remained the same or increased. A sedentary lifestyle has become so common that the majority is marching toward couch-potato status.

Nothing illustrates the effects of reduced physical activity more vividly than retirement from professional sports. For instance, TV sports channels show many superstars of yesteryear carrying extra weight.

Excess body fat positivity

Obesity and being overweight are the new normal in different regions for multiple reasons. Body positivity frequently outshouts the potential health dangers associated with excess body fat.

Being overweight is perceived as a sign of affluence, strength, and good health in most of Africa. The larger one looks, the stronger and healthier one is perceived. Slim bodies or weight loss are often associated with poor health, poverty, or a combination of the two. A "big booty" in women is attractive and sought after, and big and overweight men are said to have a "sense of presence."

There is little if any, public awareness of the statistics that show that people of African and South Asian descent develop diabetes at a much lower body mass index (BMI) than their Caucasian counterparts.

Lack of sleep and rest

Lack of sleep and rest, whether voluntary or forced, can cause a variety of health problems.

Political turmoil, economic downturn, and hopelessness can cause people to worry about what tomorrow will bring and lose sleep.

Many immigrants in Europe, America, and the Middle East have multiple menial jobs and work long hours to support themselves and family members in Africa and South Asia. Sleep and rest are often sacrificed for the millions in remittances sent home monthly.

It should be noted, though, that the link between lack of sleep, overeating, and weight gain is rarely highlighted.

Religious and spiritual belief

Illness, including symptoms of type 2 diabetes, is often attributed to a spiritual attack or witchcraft, so spiritual intervention is sought. However, no changes are made to diet or lifestyle.

Non-professional teachings and home remedies

Unverified information and teaching by self-styled gurus through social media, online platforms and word of mouth is more readily accepted than formal education programmes by healthcare professionals.

People are willing to explore home remedies over "Western medicines" and formal diabetes education.

There is no shortage of willing participants to try out instant cures that require no changes to diet or lifestyle.

Snapshot of Reasons

- Sincere belief that type 2 diabetes is inevitable.
- Carbohydrates are safe ground and are the base of every meal.
- Increased consumption of fast foods, refined grains, and high-sugar foods.
- Personal healthcare is not prioritised and is often out-sourced.
- Reduced physical activity.
- Being overweight is a sign of a good life, strength, and affluence.
- Weight loss is associated with poor health and poverty.
- Inadequate sleep and rest.
- Religious and spiritual intervention rarely calls for changes to diet and lifestyle.
- Non-professional teachings and home remedies are more readily accepted than Western medicines and structured education programmes.

Type 2 diabetes is a complex and multifaceted disease. The above list is only a subset of the reasons for the rise in the number of those afflicted with the illness.

CHAPTER 3

The Ideal: Your Body Without Diabetes

Knowing how your body works without diabetes can help you understand what has gone wrong when you get diabetes. You won't know where to start if you have no idea about how it should work.

Our bodies need energy to fuel internal functions like the heartbeat and support external activities such as walking. The primary source of energy is blood sugar. The concentration of sugar in the blood is measured in either millimoles per litre (mmol/L) or milligrams per decilitre (mg/dL).

The normal blood sugar level for a person without diabetes is between 4 and 5.4 mmol/L (72 and 99 mg/dL) before breakfast and up to 7.8 mmol/L (140 mg/dL) two hours after food (NICE). This is approximately one teaspoon of sugar.

The United Kingdom and Commonwealth countries use mmol/L whilst United Staes, Germany, and other counties use mg/dL. One mmol/L of sugar is equivalent to

18mg/dL. You can covert from either unit of measure to the other.

The pancreas, a gland that lies horizontally behind your stomach, releases one of two hormones, either insulin or glucagon, depending on the blood sugar level. Think of hormones as chemical signals

The following diagram illustrates how the pancreas regulates blood sugar.

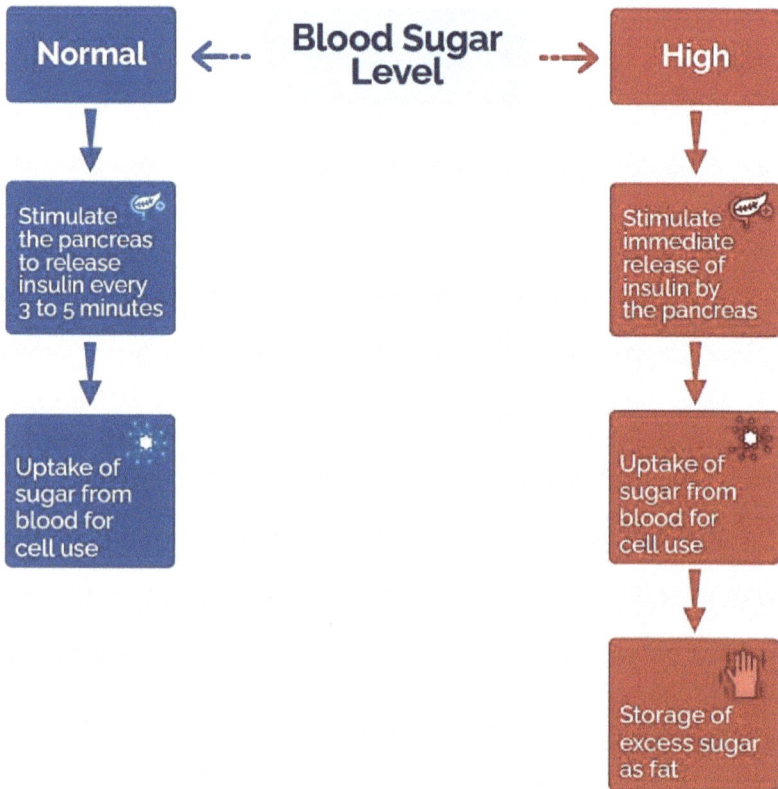

Part of the food you eat is broken down into sugar, which enters the bloodstream and gets circulated around the body. A rise in blood sugar level makes the pancreas release insulin; and insulin triggers the body to absorb

blood sugar for immediate use as energy and storage of excess, first in the liver, then as fat under the skin.

The pancreas produces insulin every three to five minutes when the blood sugar is within the normal range to fuel the brain, heartbeat, breathing, and other internal functions. So it has no downtime and constantly works to maintain blood sugar within the safe limits.

Fasting and blood sugar

The diagram below illustrates how blood sugar is regulated during fasting.

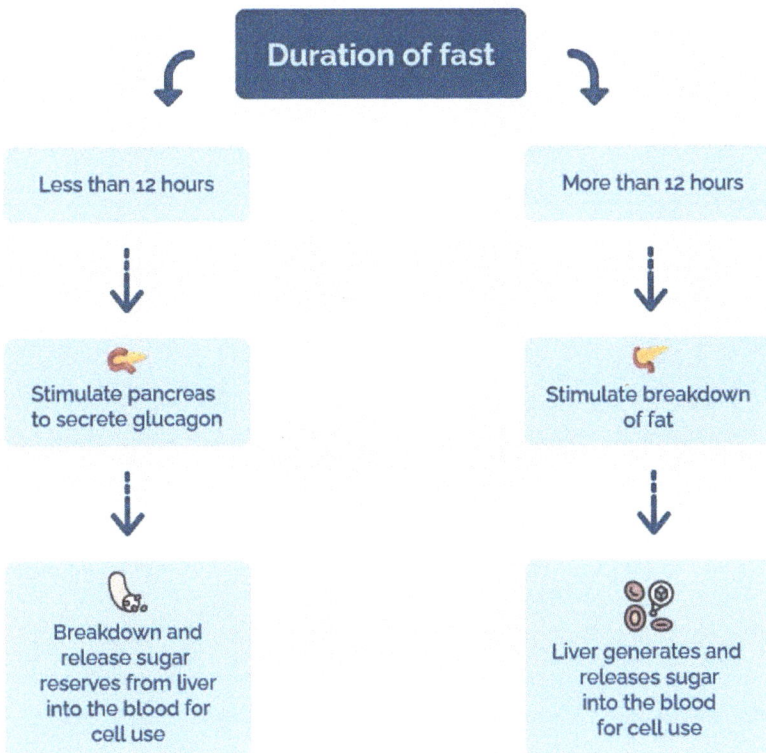

Duration of fast	
Less than 12 hours	More than 12 hours
Stimulate pancreas to secrete glucagon	Stimulate breakdown of fat
Breakdown and release sugar reserves from liver into the blood for cell use	Liver generates and releases sugar into the blood for cell use

A decrease in blood sugar below the set minimum during a short fast of less than twelve hours (for example, in between meals) induces the pancreas to release glucagon, a signal to the liver to release stored sugar.

During extended periods of fasting (more than 12 hours), after depleting sugar reserves in the liver, your body breaks down fats for energy.

So, under normal circumstances, the body's built-in intelligence effectively responds to peaks and lows of blood sugar triggered by food, physical activity, lifestyle choices, and unexpected incidents.

Summary

Normal Blood Sugars

When	Measurement	
	mmol/L	mg/dL
Before meals	4.0 to 5.4	72 to 99
2 hours after meals	up to 7.8	up to 140

Key Points

- The body primarily employs the pancreas and the liver to regulate blood sugar.
- Your blood sugar is never constant. It responds to food, physical activity, fasting, and many other factors.

Your Body Disrupted by Diabetes

What is diabetes?

Diabetes is the impairment of the body's blood sugar or glucose self-regulation system. The body is no longer able to naturally keep blood sugar at safe levels. Think of blood sugar as a fire: useful under control and can be destructive uncontrolled. The words *glucose* and *sugar* are used interchangeably in this book.

Though diabetes does not spread as quickly as a fire, the knock-on effects can lead to serious health issues. Road signs on the way to type 2 diabetes include pre-diabetes and gestational diabetes (diabetes in pregnancy).

Pre-diabetes

Pre-diabetes (or non-diabetic hyperglycaemia) is a warning sign that blood sugar levels are higher than normal but not high enough for a diagnosis of type 2 diabetes. A blood sugar level between 5.5 to 6.9 mmol/L (100 to 125 mg/dL) after at least eight hours of not eating (e.g., first thing in the morning before breakfast) falls in the pre-diabetes range.

Diet and lifestyle changes may prevent this from progressing to type 2 diabetes.

Gestational diabetes (diabetes in pregnancy)

Gestational diabetes is characterised by higher-than-normal blood sugar levels during pregnancy.

The blood sugar concentration is at least 5.6 mmol/L (100 mg/dL) or above first thing in the morning before breakfast (or after at least 8 hours of not eating) and at least 7.8 mmol/L (140mg/dL) 1 hour after a meal.

It can harm both the mother and the baby if not controlled. Thus, a combination of diet and lifestyle changes and prescribed medication can bring blood sugar to safe levels.

Though the blood sugar generally returns to its usual level after delivery, the risk of developing type 2 diabetes needs to be continually monitored and managed.

Development of type 2 diabetes

The following points describe the slow march toward the development of type 2 diabetes:
- Consistently high blood sugar induces the pancreas to produce more and more insulin. Excess sugar is stored first in the liver and then the rest of the body as fat.
- A build-up of fat, particularly around organs, blunts the body's sensitivity to insulin (commonly referred to as insulin resistance), requiring more and more to work on the same levels of blood sugar.

- A stressed and overworked pancreas eventually ceases to function optimally, so blood sugar remains higher than safe levels.
- The body may resort to employing the kidneys to dump body fluid and flush out excess blood sugar through urine. This leads to increased thirst, frequency of passing urine, and dehydration.
- Despite the high levels of blood sugar, the body may start to break down fat to meet some of its energy requirements, resulting in some weight loss.
- High blood sugar provides a breeding ground for opportunistic bacteria and creates problems like genital itching, thrush, cuts, or wounds that take longer to heal, and severe reactions to infections.
- Excess blood sugar leads to a build-up of unhealthy blood fat called cholesterol.

A blood sugar level of 7 mmol/L (126 mg/dL) or more after at least eight hours of not eating (e.g., first thing in the morning before breakfast) falls in the diabetes range.

Not everyone gets the common signs and symptoms of diabetes. Urine and blood samples are required to test for it.

Statistics show that most people only find out they have type 2 diabetes after a routine checkup for other health issues. Individuals of African, Middle Eastern, and South Asian descent are twice as likely to get type 2 diabetes at the age of 25 compared to their Caucasian counterparts, who usually develop this at 40 (Diabetes UK).

Furthermore, the Middle East has one of the fastest-growing numbers of people diagnosed with type 2 diabetes in the world (IDF).

Diagnosing diabetes

There are several tests that can be used to diagnose diabetes;

1. **A fasting blood glucose test.** Your blood glucose is checked after 8 hours of not eating.
2. **An HBA1c test.** For this test a blood sample will be taken. You don't have to fast for this test.
3. **An oral glucose tolerance test.** Your blood glucose level is measured before and two hours after drinking a liquid that contains glucose.
4. **A random blood glucose.** The blood sample is taken at any time during the day regardless of whether you have eaten or not especially if you have symptoms of a high blood sugar like increased thirst, urination and or tiredness.

Complications or problems created by diabetes

High blood sugar levels over a long period of time may lead to some of the following complications:

1. Damage to the tiny blood vessels in the back of the eyes, causing partial to full loss of sight.
2. Loss of sensation in the feet because of nerve damage, slow healing of cuts and wounds due to reduced blood circulation, and the development of ulcers that may lead to amputations.
3. Risk of heart attack and stroke because of the hardening and eventual blocking of the large blood vessels.
4. Damage to kidney blood vessel clusters that filter waste, causing high blood pressure, and the increase in pressure causing further damage to the delicate kidney filtering system.

5. Erectile dysfunction in men and loss of sensation in women due to nerve damage and reduced blood flow.
6. Increased risk of gum disease due to high sugar in the saliva.
7. Increased risk of some cancers (liver, pancreas, colon, bladder, etc.).
8. Increased risk of dementia.
9. Non-alcoholic fatty liver disease caused by a buildup of fat in the liver, impeding one of its functions of blood sugar regulation.
10. High-risk pregnancies and big babies.
11. Risk of diabetic comas

Accepting the reality

The sooner you come to terms with the reality of diabetes, the better your chances are to win the unending battle against it. Reading to this page is a big step forward. If you have been diagnosed with diabetes, you do not have to fight it alone.

Here's a list of those you might enlist to be on your team:

- Your primary care provider, a general practitioner, may manage your diabetes or refer you to specialists.
- An endocrinologist, a doctor who specialises in diabetes.
- A diabetes nurse specialist/consultant whose responsibilities include diabetes education, assessing and meeting your nutritional needs, monitoring your blood sugar, managing, and treating low and high blood sugars, and promoting self-care.

- A registered dietitian or nutrition adviser, an expert in food and nutrition, who can help you with meal planning and teach you how your food choices affect blood sugar.
- A pharmacist, an expert who can help you keep track of all your medications and explain how they work.
- A mental health provider, a social worker, a psychologist, or a psychiatrist who can teach you coping skills, help with behaviour change, and provide emotional support.

Summary

What fasting blood sugar levels mean

Measurement		Type of Diabetes
mmol/L	mg/dL	
5.5 to 6.9	100 to 125	Prediabetes
Above 5.6 *	Above 100 *	Gestational Diabetes
7.0 or above	126 or above	Type 2 Diabetes
* During pregnancy		

Key Points

- Not everyone gets the common signs and symptoms of diabetes.
- Most people find out they have pre-diabetes or diabetes during routine health checkups.
- High blood sugar levels put the body at risk of various illnesses and complications.
- Blood tests for diagnosing diabetes must be done in a qualified lab, not at a health fair or by using a blood glucose meter.
- Enlist and follow the advice of your healthcare provider to manage and prevent complications.

CHAPTER 5

Choosing Your Lane

I t is not uncommon for the newly diagnosed to feel that it is the end of "normal" life. Most who have never been tested do not think they have a role to play in the diabetes arena.

This chapter covers four options or lanes from which you can choose the direction you want to go, namely, prevention, remission, managing, or uncontrolled. Unless you select your preferred option, you may find yourself in the most inconvenient lane that leads to the unwanted outcomes and complications discussed in the last chapter.

Lane 1: Prevention

The well-known quote "Prevention is better than cure" is as applicable to type 2 diabetes as it is to any other disease. Contrary to what some may think, diabetes is not inevitable even in old age. Moreover, a family history of diabetes or gestational diabetes isn't a life sentence for you either.

Anyone with the know-how has a fighting chance of preventing it. Prevention is a lifetime commitment; it is a lane to living well.

Lane 2: Remission/Reversal

Pre-diabetes is reversible (remission) and so is type 2 diabetes. Unfortunately, countless people only find out they have diabetes after complications have set in. Some choose to be in denial and live in the hope that it will go away as silently as it came. But it never does.

It is essential to be tested and know your status. Acceptance of your condition is the first step. The next is to commit to reversing it. You will need help and support from both family and healthcare professionals.

Lane 3: Managing diabetes

Having diabetes doesn't mean the end of life. It can be managed with the help and support of healthcare professionals and family. Well-managed type 2 diabetes can either evade complications or stop further deterioration.

Lane 4: Uncontrolled diabetes

Having an occasional high blood sugar level is not the same as having consistently high blood sugar levels all day every day. Uncontrolled blood sugar levels can damage parts of your body and lead to health complications.

The way forward

Most people can change tracks on the four-lane motorway described above. Some may start in the managing or uncontrolled lane and cross into the remission lane. Accordingly, the end of the remission lane joins the prevention track.

As diabetes is multi-faceted, you may need a combination of actions or changes to achieve your goals, whichever lane you choose. The rest of this book is dedicated to helping you reach your goal.

CHAPTER 6

Let Food Be Thy Medicine

The familiar quote "Let food be thy medicine and let medicine be thy food" demands basic knowledge and understanding of what you eat. This chapter reveals the recommended quantities (doses) to support good health, discusses current amounts generally consumed and their effect on blood sugar, and gives pointers to how you should eat. This is not a sprint with a finishing line; rather, this is an integral part of a healthy lifestyle.

Eating for optimal health

All medicines have a purpose, recommended quantities, how often they need to be taken, and side effects. Not following prescription instructions may limit the benefit of medicines and risk health deterioration.

You may wonder what the purpose of food is besides satisfying hunger. The complete list is beyond the scope of this book. Some of the needs your body is designed to meet from food are listed below:

– Provide energy
– Enable waste removal
– Strengthen bones and bolster immunity

- Build and repair tissues and muscles
- Lubricate joints and facilitate movement

The following plate is an indicator of the recommended portions and quantities of food for a person without diabetes.

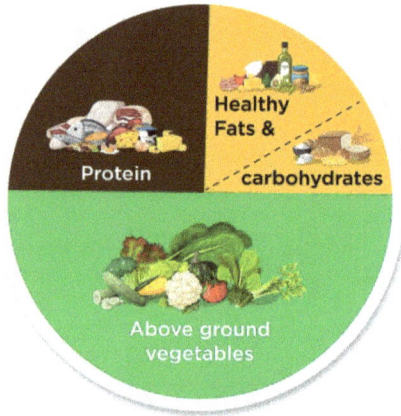

Half the plate is made up of aboveground vegetables (kale, cabbage, broccoli, etc.); a quarter of proteins (beef, lamb, chicken, fish, eggs, tofu, etc.); and the remaining quarter is made up of a combination of healthy fats (avocado, full-fat dairy, coconut oil, etc.) and carbohydrates (grain products and starchy foods).

How the majority eats

Carbohydrates (carbs) make up more than 60% of the diet for the majority. The largest portion of every meal is either starchy foods (potatoes, cassava, sweet potatoes, and yams) or refined cereals (wheat, maize, rice, millet, and sorghum). Children in parts of the world are taught from an early age to consume more carbs and resist cravings for protein.

Protein and vegetables are mostly cooked in super-refined cooking oil or man-made fats. The plate below is an example of what many consider "normal eating."

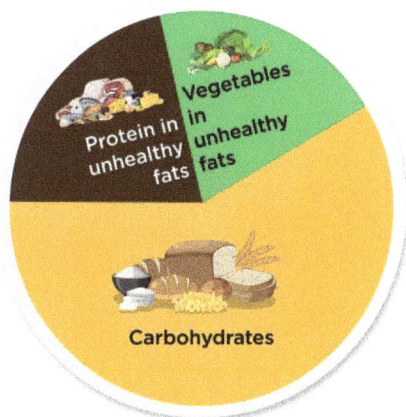

Impact on blood sugar

Many diabetes patients are baffled when they find out their blood sugar is high. "But I don't eat sugar" is a recurring protest. "I have changed my whole diet and stopped eating white bread and white rice and replaced it with brown bread and brown rice. I don't understand where the sugar is coming from."

They learn the body breaks down carbohydrates or starchy foods (termed hard foods in the West Indies) into sugar. Many think that whole-meal bread does not put the blood sugar up, but three slices of whole-meal bread contain approximately 10 teaspoons of sugar.

The following table shows an estimate of the number of teaspoons of sugar in a standard serving of carbohydrates.

Food	Serving (grams)	Teaspoons of sugar
Wholemeal Spaghetti	90	18
Chapatti/Roti	180	16
Cooked rice	200	13
Pap (from maize meal)	175	10
Wholemeal Bread x 3 slices	120	10

Common snacks in between meals increase the percentage of carbohydrates consumed daily. The table below lists the approximate sugar content in common snacks.

Food	Serving (grams)	Teaspoons of sugar
Baklawa	180	19
Potato Crisps	150	18
Maamoul	150	17
Fat cook/ Puff puff	140	14
Bhajia/ Pakora	210	9
Plantain Crisps	75	9
Samosa Vegetable	120	7

You can imagine the extra effort your body has to put in to bring down the blood sugar to the safe level of approximately one teaspoon, a blood sugar concentration between 4.0 to 5.4 mmol/L (72 to 99 mg/dL).

Planning a healthy plate

Making food medicine does not happen by itself; and knowledge, on its own, isn't enough. A review of the food you are eating will go a long way to helping you achieve your goals. Putting into practice what you now know will make a difference. The following few ground rules put you in good stead:

- Eat foods as close to their natural state as possible.
- Reduce added sugars like honey, molasses, jaggery, table sugar, and syrup.
- Reduce refined grains like super-refined maize meal, white flour, and white chapatti flour.

Control of portions is key. It helps if you plan your plate around what you enjoy eating. The following four steps are recommended:

Step 1: First on the plate are aboveground vegetables.

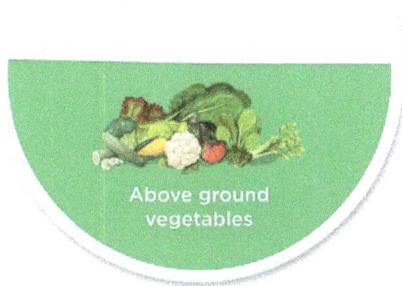

Allocate half the plate to vegetables that grow above the ground like kale, cabbage, spinach, rape, saag, tomatoes, salad greens, and courgettes (baby marrow). They are high in vitamins and fibre. For maximum benefits and retention of nutrients, minimise the cooking time, the temperature, and the liquid.

The table below lists examples of vegetables that grow above the ground.

Low Starchy Vegetables		
Ackee	Celery	Rape/Saag
Artichoke	Cherry Tomatoes	Sugar Snap Peas
Asparagus	Chow Chow / chayote	Rocket
Aubergine	Cucumber	Spinach
Baby Corn	Edamame	Mustard Greens
Bamboo Shoots	Garden Peas	Sweet Potato Leaves
Broccoli	Green Beans	Sweet Peppers
Brussel Sprouts	Hibiscus leaves	Swiss Chard
Butternut Squash	Edamame	Mushrooms
Cauliflower	Okra varieties	Pumpkin

Many of us are creatures of habit and stick to the same vegetables. Challenge yourself and try something new every week. The wider the variety of vegetables you eat, the higher the mix of nutrients you give your body.

Step 2: Add protein.

Fill a quarter of your plate with protein-rich foods like beef, lamb, fish, eggs, lentils, beans, etc.

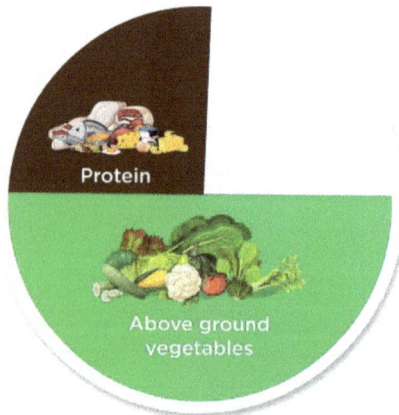

The portion should be no bigger than the size of your palm (the inner surface of the hand that extends between the wrist to the base of the fingers).

Good quality proteins include the following:

Animal Proteins	Plant Proteins
Eggs	Nuts
Fish	Seeds
Chicken	*Beans/ Lentils
Beef	Wholegrains
Game	Hemp
Edible insects	Tofu
Kefir/Sour Milk/Yoghurt/Cheese	Tempeh

* *Although lentils, beans, and quinoa contain protein, they are also high in carbohydrates. Hence, the quantity of other carbs like bread, rice, or chapatti should be proportionally reduced.*

Step 3: Add healthy fats and carbohydrates.

Fill the remaining quarter with healthy fats and carbohydrates.

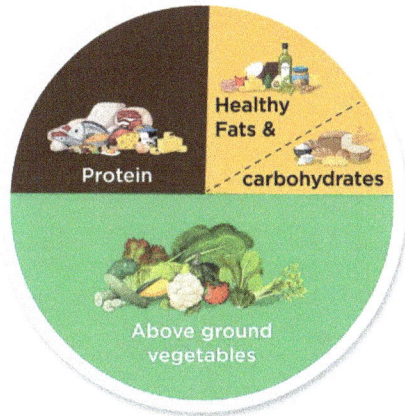

Healthy fats like avocado, olive oil, butter, and coconut oil help the body to absorb fat-soluble vitamins like A, D, and E. Contrary to common perception, healthy fats are good for you. Studies have shown that increasing natural fats in your diet helps to promote a sense of fullness and lowers bad cholesterol.

The table below lists some healthy fats.

Recommended Fats			
Oils		**Full Fat Dairy**	
Goose fat	Olive oil	Greek Style Yoghurt	Cream
Lard	Palm oil	Whole milk	Grass-fed butter
Peanut oil	Hemp oil	Ghee	Cheese
Coconut oil	Rapeseed oil	**Alternative Milk**	
Avocado oil	Pumpkin seed oil	Almond	Cashew
Flaxseed oil		**Seeds, nuts and nut butters**	
Fish/ Eggs/Meat		Almond	Brazil
Anchovies	Kapenta	Cashew	Peanut
Mackerel	Sardines	Pistachio	Walnut
Salmon	Trout	**Other**	
Free Range Eggs	Grass-fed meat	Olives	Avocado

Fats to minimise consumption include the following:

Fats to minimise	
Vegetable oils	Corn oil
Canola oil	Cottonseed oil
Safflower oil	Soybean oil
Sunflower oil	Margarines

Trans fats, used to make most cakes, biscuits, and fried foods, raise bad cholesterol.

Last on the plate are carbohydrates (starchy foods and cereals). They include rice, lentils, potatoes, sweet potatoes, maize meal, plantain, green bananas, millet, and beans.

So, the portion of carbohydrates should be less than a quarter of the plate. The tables below list examples of carbohydrates.

Breads, Cereals and Grains (White or Wholemeal)	Beans & Lentils
Bread	Beans (kidney, navy, pinto)
Bagel	Lentils
Tortilla or pitta bread	Baked beans
English muffin	Refried beans
Chapatti/ Roti	Hummus
Rice	Split Peas
Pasta	Chickpeas
Bulgur Wheat	Soya beans
Couscous	Black Turtle Beans
Quinoa	Butter Beans
High Starchy Vegetables	**Starchy Flours**
Breadfruit	Gari
Corn	Maize Meal
Potato	Millet Flour
Sweet potato	Besan
Yam	Ground Rice
Green Banana	Kenkey
Plantain	Cassava
Taro	Sorghum
Eddoes	Teff
Cassava	Ondhwa

A word about "diabetic foods"

Products labelled "diabetic food" in stores and supermarkets have as much sugar as their ordinary varieties. Avoid them. You are better off sticking to natural foods.

What should I eat?

It is a recurring question when countless people learn about food and its effects on blood sugar. The answer is simple: You plan your meals around what you like eating, stick to natural whole foods, and be mindful of their effect on blood sugar.

 The following guide of what to eat more and less at breakfast contrasts with how the majority currently eat.

Meal	Eat and drink more	Eat and drink less
Breakfast	• Fish • Non-processed meats • Eggs • Berries • Full fat yoghurt, cheese, milk • Nut milks (homemade if possible) • Water, Tea and Coffee	• Bread • Chapatti • Rice • Maize meal porridge or Grits • Sausages • Cereals (Granola, Corn or Bran flakes) • High-sugar fruits • Condensed Milk • Sugar, Honey, Molasses or Sweeteners • Fruit juice (sweetened or unsweetened)

A high-carb breakfast dramatically increases your blood sugar, and the corresponding blood sugar dip is likely to make you crave a high-sugar snack by mid-morning.

Good-quality protein and healthy fats will help steady your blood sugars all morning. If you are used to having a high-carb breakfast, be kind to yourself and reduce it gradually to reprogramme your mind and palate.

✳✳✳

Now that you know that the "healthy lunch" you have had all your life isn't that good for you, change is due. This is not a suggestion to ditch "staple foods" but rather a call to minimise what the body considers as excess to needs.

Meal	Eat and drink more	Eat and drink less
Lunch	• Meat • Beans • Lentils • Cauliflower Rice • Ghee • Lard • Coconut oil • Palm oil • Water, Fermented Drinks (Kombucha), Tea & Coffee	• Pap (Sadza, Ugali, Amala, Gari) Idli, Injera • Rice • Bread • Chapatti • Takeaway foods • Pasta • Potatoes • Yam • Plantain • Colas, Super Malt, Alcohol, Energy Drinks, Fruit Squashes (with or no added sugar)

The major change should be in reducing portion sizes of starchy foods such as injera, sadza, gari, and chapatti and eating moderate amounts of good-quality proteins.

Having more vegetables will help you feel full as they are a good source of fibre. Including healthy fats in your meals will give you a sense of fullness and slow down the uptake of sugar into the blood.

***

Try to eat your dinner two to four hours before bedtime. It gives your body ample time to digest food and reduces the risk of sleep disruption.

Meal	Eat and drink more	Eat and drink less
Dinner	• Meat • Beans • Lentils • Cauliflower Rice • Ghee • Lard • Coconut oil • Palm oil • Water, Fermented Drinks (Kombucha), Tea & Coffee	• Pap (Sadza,Ugali,Amala, Gari) Idli, Injera • Rice • Bread • Chapatti • Takeaway foods • Pasta • Potatoes • Yam • Plantain • Colas, Super Malt, Alcohol, Energy Drinks, Fruit Squashes (with or no added sugar)

Base your dinner on low-starchy vegetables and follow the plate guide discussed earlier. Avoid foods and drinks that are likely to increase your blood sugar.

***

Try to avoid snacking, but if you need to, stick to the recommended list and be mindful of quantities.

A boiled egg or one and a half tablespoons of raw nuts or seeds can satisfy your hunger in between meals. Another good option is fresh berries with full-fat yoghurt with no added sugar.

Meal	Eat and drink more	Eat and drink less
Snacks	• Raw nuts and seeds • Full fat yoghurt • Vegetable sticks like carrot or celery • A small piece of cheese (no bigger than your middle finger) • A boiled egg	• High sugar fruits (like grapes, bananas) • Fried foods • Sweet potatoes • Colas

Takeaways

– All starchy foods increase blood sugar.
– Make vegetables that grow above the ground the base of your meals.
– Eat moderate protein, no more than the size of the palm of your hand.
– Increase natural fats (not man-made).
– Eat foods as close to their natural state as possible.

- Reduce added sugars like honey, molasses, jaggery, table sugar, and syrup.
- If possible, avoid snacking.

CHAPTER 7

What About Fruits?

"Fruits are nature's candy" is a popular quote that highlights the sweetness of fruits. Though wild and cultivated fruits are often put in the same basket, there are notable differences. For example, the apple that grows in the wild is different from cultivated varieties.

Wild fruits are generally small in size, high in fibre, have large seeds, have a small amount of fruit flesh, and have low levels of sugar. On the other hand, cultivated fruits are bigger, some are seedless, have more fruit flesh, and most are typically high in sugar.

Taste (high sugar content) and the ability to withstand shipping are some of the main factors that determine which fruits and varieties are on supermarket shelves.

Sugar content in fruit

The sweeter the fruit, the more sugar it contains.

The table below shows how much sugar is in some popular fruits.

Fruit	Serving	Teaspoons of sugar
Figs	1 cup	7
Lychees	1 cup	6
Banana	1 Large	5
Mango	1 Large	5
Persimmon	1 fruit	4
Dates	3 fruits	3

It is not immediately apparent that one large banana can contain up to five teaspoons of sugar and one persimmon approximately four.

Benefits of fruits

Fruits can be part of a healthy diet when eaten in moderation. Benefits include the following:

- Some are high in vitamin C, which supports the immune system and keeps teeth and gums healthy. Fruits with high vitamin C content include oranges and strawberries.
- Some are good sources of fibre, which aids regular bowel movement and can help lower cholesterol levels. High-fibre fruits include apples, pears, blackberries, and raspberries.
- Fruits high in potassium, like bananas and mangos, help maintain healthy blood pressure and regulate fluid balance in the body.
- Fruits that are high in folate, like oranges and mangos, help the body produce red blood cells and support healthy foetal development.

- Fruits that are rich in antioxidants, like black plums, prunes, and berries, help fight off illness and can protect the skin.

You may wonder how you can get the benefits of fruit without the cost of high sugar. The table below lists fresh fruits that contain less sugar.

Fruit	Serving (1 cup)	Teaspoons of sugar
Blueberries	1	3
Mulberries	1	2
Loganberries	1	2
Strawberries	1	1 ½
Blackberries	1	1 ½
Cranberries	1	1
Raspberries	1	1

Dried fruits vs. fresh fruits

Dried fruits contain significantly higher amounts of sugar than the fresh varieties. The reduction of water content in dried fruit concentrates the sugar.

You, therefore, need to be mindful of the quantities you consume and the potential effect on blood sugar. The table below shows how much sugar is in some dried fruits.

Dried fruit	Serving	Teaspoons of sugar
Raisins	1 cup	17
Cranberries	1 cup	14
Figs	1 fruit	2

Tips

✓ **Do**

1. Familiarise yourself with fruits that contain a lot of sugar.
2. Choose fruits that contain less sugar, especially berries (e.g., blueberries, raspberries, or strawberries).
3. Have fruit with something fatty like a small piece of cheese, full-fat yoghurt, or a tablespoon of raw nuts like almonds, peanuts, or walnuts.
4. Have fruit after a balanced meal. It slows down the uptake of sugar.

✗ **Don't**

1. Eat fruits that contain a lot of sugar.
2. Eat large amounts of fruit.
3. Eat fruit in between meals as it will be digested quicker and increase your blood sugar.
4. Put a lot of fruit and or fruit juice into smoothies.

CHAPTER 8

Drinks

This chapter explores types of beverages, how they affect your blood sugars and healthy drink options.

Alcohol

Most of the questions on drinks relate to alcohol. Effect on blood sugars depends on many factors, including the type of alcoholic drink, mixers, and when you had your last meal.

- **Alcoholic drinks with no sugar**

Most spirits (hard alcohols) do not have sugar, so they do not raise the blood sugar level. Common types include:

o   tequila,
o   whiskey,
o   vodka,
o   gin,
o   brandy.

The type of mixer can make the drink high in sugar.

- **Alcoholic drinks with sugar**

Sugar content in alcoholic drinks varies considerably. All beers contain sugar and so do liqueurs, fortified wines, sherries, cider, and pre-mixed drinks.

The table below shows approximate quantities of sugar in some alcoholic drinks.

Drink	Serving	Teaspoons of sugar
Cider (sweet, 5% *ABV)	1 pint	5
Beer (4.6% *ABV)	1 pint	3
White Wine (Sweet)	250ml	3
Stout (4% *ABV)	1 pint	2
Sweet Liqueur	25ml	1 ½
White Wine (Dry)	250ml	½

ABV Alcohol by volume

In the UK most wines do not have a label showing how much sugar is in them as this is not required by law, but many wines contain considerable amounts of sugar.

- **Delayed response to low blood sugar (hypoglycaemia or hypo)**

All types of alcohol can delay the response to a low blood sugar level because the liver prioritises filtering alcohol above releasing stored sugar into the bloodstream. This means that you run the risk of having a dangerously low blood sugar level if you drink alcohol and take medicines that lower blood sugar.

- **Tips if you choose to drink (and have diabetes)**

o Ask your healthcare provider about how to drink safely.

o   Do not drink on an empty stomach.
o   Do not drink too much.
o   Be on the lookout for signs of low blood sugar (hypo).
o   Make sure your friends and family can recognise a hypo.
o   Check your blood sugar regularly.

Non-alcoholic drinks

- **High-sugar drinks**

Freshly squeezed juice (homemade or shop-bought) is very high in sugar. You need at least five to six oranges or apples to make a glass of fruit juice. Blending causes the sugars contained within the fruit to be more readily available as you drink. Your blood sugar level is likely to dramatically go up. Have the fruit instead or dilute the fruit juice one part to three or four parts of water.

Soft drinks, energy drinks, and squashes still contain a lot of sugar despite efforts by governments the world over to have the amounts of sugar reduced.

High-sugar drinks include the following:

Drink	Serving (ml)	Teaspoons of sugar
Condensed Milk	150	17
Super Malt	330	10
Apple Juice	330	7
Orange Juice	330	7
Cola	330	7
Mango Lassi	250	6

- **Non-Alcoholic Beers**

Contrary to perception non-alcoholic beers do not always contain less sugar. A 330ml can of non-alcoholic beer can contain up to 3 teaspoons of sugar.

- **Hot drinks**

Most ready-made lattes and chocolate drinks contain considerable amounts of sugar as shown in the table below.

Hot drink	Serving (ml)	Teaspoons of sugar
Hot Chocolate	475	10
Caffe Mocha	475	6
Latte	475	4
Cappuccino	475	2 ½
Espresso	60	0
Coffee (black)	475	0
Tea (black)	475	0

Unless you add sugar to espresso, black coffee, or black tea, they won't increase your blood sugar.

- **Artificially sweetened drinks (diet drinks)**

There is ongoing research into how diet drinks and drinks with artificial sweeteners affect blood sugar. Some diabetic patients have found out that these drinks raise their blood sugar levels and make them crave sugar.

- **Water**

The best drink is plain water. Roughly 60% of your body is water. Consequently, your body needs enough water to function properly, which includes aiding digestion, regulating body temperature, removing waste, and carrying nutrients and oxygen around the body.

It is essential to drink enough water to meet your unique needs, which depend on factors such as age, health, size, activity levels, type of job, and the climate of where you live. Drinking little and often is the best way to stay hydrated. Several thinktanks recommend drinking at least two litres of water per day.

Try adding a few slices of cucumber, fresh mint, or lemon for an added boost if drinking plain water is a challenge for you.

Takeaways

– Reduce intake of alcohol.
– Reduce intake of high-sugar drinks.
– Drink more water.

CHAPTER 9

Physical Activity

What it means to be physically active varies from person to person. In a nutshell, it is sitting down less and moving your body more. This chapter explores recommendations, types, barriers, and ways to increase physical activity.

Recommendations

The minimum recommended for a person with diabetes or at risk of diabetes is 30 minutes of physical activity a day at least five times a week. Walking counts as an activity.

The benefits include the following:

- It helps to lower blood sugar.
- It aids digestion by increasing blood flow to the stomach.
- It strengthens bones and improves bone density and balance.
- It may help block negative thoughts or distract from daily worries.

Types of physical activity

Types of activities you can add include the following:

- Walking, whether indoors or outdoors, can be effective in reducing blood sugar levels.
- Yoga encourages strength, flexibility, and relaxation.
- High-intensity interval training can reduce blood pressure and burn fat.
- Incidental exercise or daily activities like gardening, housework, going up the stairs, and dancing also count.

Common hindrances to physical activity

The list below includes some of the reasons people are less active.

- The environment (climate extremes, no sidewalks, etc.) restricts outside activities.
- Making a living is prioritised above physical activity.
- Mobility issues caused by leg or back pain, and other ailments.
- Minimal activity is perceived as a sign of "good living."
- Cycling or walking to work is looked down upon in parts of Africa and South Asia.

Ways to increase physical activity

There is no one-size-fits-all. Do what works for you to incorporate physical activity into every aspect of your life. You may consider the following tips:

- Join a gym or a walking group if you need the motivation of being in a class.
- Get the right equipment and instruction if you prefer to exercise indoors on your own.

- Don't drive everywhere. Walk where you can or use public transport.
- Get off the bus or train one or two stops before the right one.
- Take a walk after a meal.
- Get a dog that you will need to walk.
- Take the stairs instead of an elevator.
- Run up the stairs instead of walking if you can.
- Try swimming if you can't walk.

CHAPTER 10

Rest, Relaxation, and Sleep

R est, relaxation, and sleep are often thought to mean the same thing. The basic definitions below draw the lines in between:

Rest: Stop working or movement.

Relaxation: Being free from tension or anxiety.

Sleep: The body is not active and there is a complete or partial suspension of consciousness.

This chapter explores how the three promote overall well-being and help to control blood sugar levels.

Rest

Time-out to rest can be either voluntary at convenient times or forced by untimely ill-health. The body cannot go on forever. It is critical to regularly unplug from a busy world.

Benefits include the following:

- Increased energy levels
- Greater productivity
- Lower stress levels

Relaxation

Experts have identified stress as one of the biggest obstacles to sleep and rest. Make every effort to manage your stress levels and seek help if it is getting in the way of normal life.

Taking time out to engage in activities that you enjoy reduces stress levels. Here are a few suggestions:

- Reading
- Walking leisurely
- Meeting up with friends and family
- Attending a club
- Maintaining what you call "me" time
- Keeping a gratitude journal
- Practicing mindfulness
- Meditating

Sleep

Lack of sleep increases hormones that stimulate appetite and promote weight gain. It has been linked to higher blood sugar levels and the development of type 2 diabetes.

There is no one-size-fits-all for the sleep each one of us needs. Some experts give a time range, and some say it is more about the quality than the quantity of sleep that matters. The bottom line is that you must get the sleep you need.

The benefits of good quality sleep include the following:

- Reduction in stress
- Improved focus and concentration
- Better weight management
- Improved immune system
- Reduced risk of health problems like diabetes

Some causes of sleep disturbances are listed below:

- Stress
- Irregular sleeping patterns from shift work
- Snacking just before bed
- Hormonal imbalance due to menopause

Useful tips to improve the quality of your sleep

- Sleep and wake up at a similar time every day if your schedule allows it.
- Ditch snacks just before bed. Drink water or have a small protein snack if you must eat.
- Avoid or limit caffeine and alcohol in the evening.
- Dim lights in your bedroom and stop using your phone and other electronic devices at least two hours before bed.
- Increase physical activity during the day.
- Practice yoga before bed.
- Make sure the temperature is cooler in your bedroom.

CHAPTER 11

Understanding Your Health Dashboard

Diabetes complications covered in Chapter 4 do not occur overnight. Catching the signs early is key to prevention; hence, the need to take control of your healthcare. If you are not in the driver's seat, there is no driver. Unlike a vehicle, healthcare cannot be parked; It keeps moving.

A responsible vehicle driver pays attention to the dashboard, understands what warning lights mean, and proactively avoids a breakdown or engine failure. Likewise, your body has health warning signals—some apparent and others not so obvious.

The expression "If you can't measure it, you can't manage it," credited to Peter Drucker, is just as applicable to healthcare as it is to management. One of the key steps toward assuming responsibility for your healthcare is to understand what is measurable and the implications of the numbers.

A combination of blood tests, urine tests, and a physical examination provide pointers to your current state of health and paint a picture of what is going well, what needs urgent attention, and warnings for what requires improvement, as illustrated in the sample dashboard below.

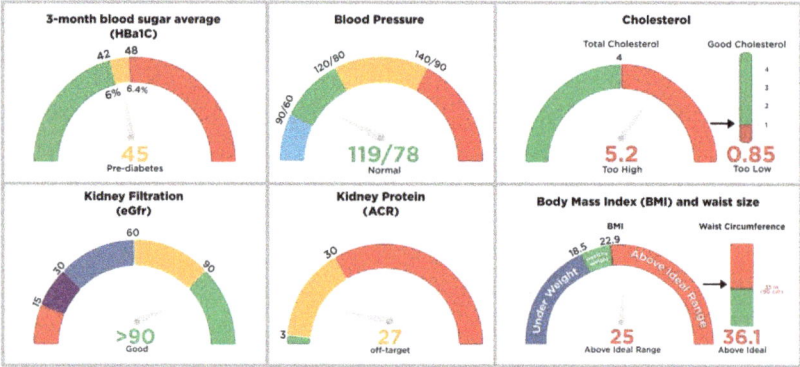

Three-month blood sugar average (HbA1c)

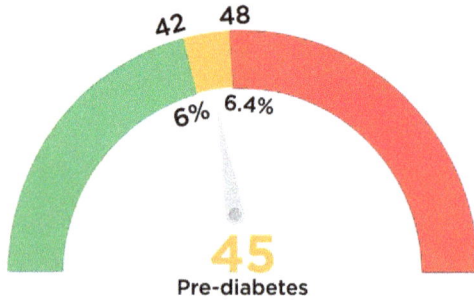

Your average blood sugar level over the last two to three months, obtained through a blood test, is measured in millimoles per mol (mmol/mol) or expressed as a percentage (%).

Measurement (mmol/mol)	Result	Measurement (%)
Less than 42	No Diabetes	Less than 6%
42 – 47	Pre-diabetes	6.0% to 6.4%
More than 48	Diabetes	More than 6.4%

It is not only a useful measure to keep an eye on, but it also informs you which lane you are in, as listed in the table above.

The pre-diabetes range is such a small window it does not take much to cross lanes. For people with diabetes, the higher the number, the bigger the risk of complications.

Blood pressure (BP)

Blood pressure is the force of circulating blood against the walls of blood vessels. Your heart is the primary organ of the circulatory system whose functions include pumping blood to other parts of the body and maintaining blood pressure.

Blood pressure is measured in millimeters of mercury (mmHg) and gives two numbers, as shown in the sample chart below.

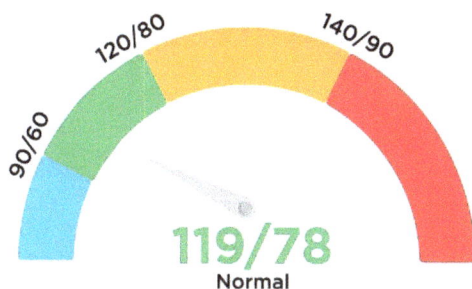

The upper number (systolic) is the pressure in the heart when it is contracting, and the lower number (diastolic) is the pressure when the heart is filling/ resting between beats.

Your healthcare provider will guide you and set your blood pressure target, taking into consideration your age and state of health.

Blood pressure classifications are shown in the following table.

Systolic BP (mmHg)	Diastolic BP (mmHg)	Classification
Below 120	Below 80	Normal
120-129	Below 80	Elevated
130-139	or 80-89	Stage 1 High BP
140 or higher	90 or higher	Stage 2 High BP

Ratio of total cholesterol to good cholesterol

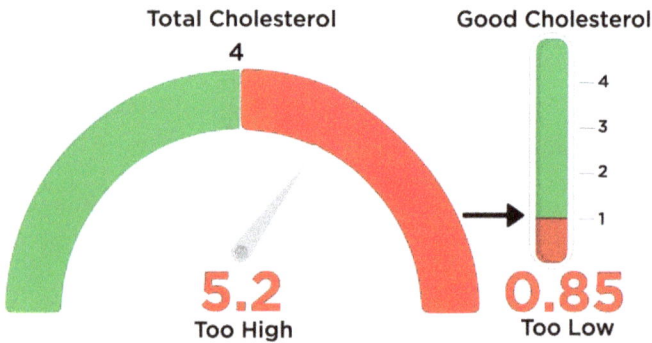

Total Cholesterol
4

Good Cholesterol

4
3
2
1

5.2
Too High

0.85
Too Low

Contrary to perception, the body needs cholesterol (blood fat), a waxy substance found in the blood. Its functions include building cells and producing hormones.

But not all cholesterol is good as inferred. The bad ones, low-density lipoprotein (LDL) and triglycerides, are some of the main predictors of heart disease and give all cholesterol a bad name.

A blood test or lipid panel provides the types and levels of cholesterol measured in millimoles per litre of blood (mmol/L) or milligrams per deciliter (mg/dL). The objective is to minimise bad cholesterol and have a higher percentage of good cholesterol.

People diagnosed with diabetes are at risk of developing heart disease and other complications.

The tables below indicates the recommended levels for people with diabetes.

Type	Level (mmol/L)	Level (mg/dL)
Total Cholesterol	below 4	below 155
Non-HDL	below 3	below 116
Good Cholesterol (HDL)	above 1	above 40
Bad Cholesterol (LDL)	below 4	below 155

Triglycerides

When	Level (mmol/L)	Level (mg/dL)
Fasting	below 1.7	below 150
Non-fasting	below 2.3	below 204

Kidney filtration (eGfr)

The filtration rate (eGFr) measures how well your kidneys are working. The tiny filters in the kidneys allow waste products to be removed from the blood while preventing the loss of important proteins and blood cells. There are five categories of kidney function, only the lower three are of any concern, as illustrated in the following chart.

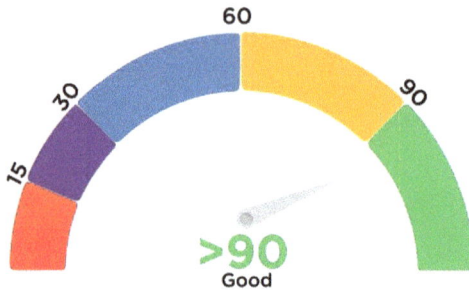

>90
Good

A blood test estimates how much waste passes through kidney filters per minute (ml/min). The table below shows what the results mean.

Level (ml/min)	Result
Greater than 90	Normal
60 – 89	Mildly decreased
30 – 59	Off target
15 – 29	Low
Less than 15	Almost all function lost

Urine protein level (Urine ACR)

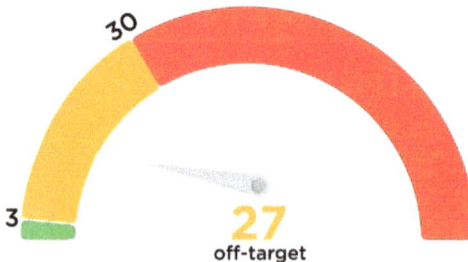

27
off-target

An albumin-creatinine ratio (ACR) test checks for signs that protein is leaking into the urine. A very low protein level means the kidneys are working well. Moderate levels may be an indicator of early stages of kidney disease, and higher levels indicate kidney disease, as shown in the results table below.

Level (mg/mmol)	Result
Less than 3	Good
Between 3 and 30	Off target
More than 30	High

Body fat

The body mass index (BMI) is a measure of body fat. The calculation, based on your height and weight, shows if you are the right weight for your height. Your waist size provides a pointer to where the body fat is stored and the type of fat buildup around your organs.

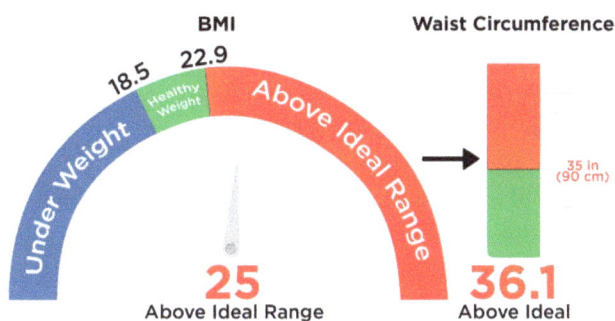

Higher levels of fat buildup in and around organs are linked to diabetes, high blood fat levels, and high blood pressure.

Though a BMI of 25 is in the healthy weight range for Caucasians, statistics show that it is above the ideal for people of African and South Asian descent who tend to be at risk of diabetes at a lower body mass index (BMI). The BMI has some drawbacks, especially in people with higher amounts of muscle; hence, waist circumference is used to assess the level of risk.

The table below reflects the level of risk associated with waist circumference for men and women of African and South Asian descent.

Men	Result	Women
Below 90cm (35.4in)	Low risk	Below 80cm (31.5in)
90cm (35.4in) and above	High risk	80cm (31.5in) and above

The numbers in the table demonstrate that there is little wiggle room in the amount of body fat you can carry.

Takeaways

– You must keep an eye on your health status, whether you have diabetes or not.
– Familiarise yourself with the numbers and what they mean.
– Find out from your healthcare provider what you need to do to stay within the recommended parameters. Your annual diabetes review is a good time to start.
– Do not walk blindly toward complications.

CHAPTER 12

Digital Devices

Thanks to technology, you can monitor your blood sugar at home, at work, at school, or on the go. Blood sugar meters (monitors) and continuous glucose monitors (CGM) measure the concentration of sugar in the blood. Monitoring gives you an idea of how your blood sugar levels respond to food, exercise, medicines, stress, and other factors.

Anyone can use the meters or monitors as part of the tools to either manage or prevent type 2 diabetes. These tools put you in the driver's seat and enable you to choose your lane with ease.

Blood sugar meters (monitors)

A blood glucose meter is a portable device that requires a disposable test strip to be inserted into it. You prick the side of your finger to release a small drop of blood, which you put on the test strip. The meter then analyses how much sugar is in the blood and displays the result on the screen in either mmol/L or mg/dL.

There are different brands of blood glucose meters. You may need to purchase this for yourself, and your healthcare provider can help you choose the one that might benefit you the most.

Continuous glucose monitors (CGM)

A CGM is a wearable device that measures your blood sugar levels throughout the day and night. A small sensor that is inserted under the skin on your arm or tummy sends blood sugar level data to a smartphone or another device.

You can swim, shower, and exercise with it and get your blood sugars without finger pricking. Some brands have customisable alerting systems that trigger notifications when the blood sugar level is too high or too low.

The best times to test/read your blood sugar level are:

- After a fasting period, usually before breakfast
- Just before food
- One to two hours after your meal
- Before bed
- Before and after exercise
- Before driving, during your journey, and when you reach your destination.

Your healthcare provider is best placed to advise you on the best times to test for you. It is helpful to keep a log of your test results, particularly if you are on medicines that can cause low blood sugar.

A food/activity diary and blood sugar log, like the one below, can help you record and monitor your activities and what you eat and the effects on your blood sugar.

Food/activity diary and blood sugar log example				
Date	Time	Blood Sugar before food/activity	Food /activity	Blood Sugar after activity or 2 hours after food
Jul 4	08:00	10	Cardio exercise	8.1
Jul 4	09:00	7.9	Porridge and sweetener	16.7
Jul 4	13:00	8.4	2 boiled eggs and water	6.0
Jul 4	18:00	5.6	Spaghetti Bolognese, coleslaw, sweetcorn	11.0
Jul 4	23:00	8.6	Bedtime	n/a

Normal and diabetic blood sugar ranges

The normal blood sugar levels for healthy individuals are:

- between 4.0 and 5.4 mmol/L (72 and 99 mg/dL) before meals and
- up to 7.8 mmol/L (140 mg/dL) two hours after eating.

The blood sugar level targets for people with type 2 diabetes are:

- between 4.0 and 7.0 mmol/L (72 and 126 mg/dL) before meals and
- under 8.5 mmol/L (153 mg/dL) two hours after eating.

Your healthcare provider may give you individualised targets after considering your age and any other illnesses or conditions you may have.

Difference between HbA1c and blood sugar level

As discussed in Chapter 11, HbA1c is the average of your blood sugar levels over the last three months. It is measured in mmol/mol or expressed as a percentage.

The concentration of sugar in your blood (obtained via a finger prick test or continuous glucose monitor) fluctuates throughout the day. It is expressed in mmol/L or mg/dL.

You can calculate the estimated HbA1c from fasting blood sugar levels. Your healthcare provider can give you pointers to the best online calculator to use.

Case studies

What can you learn from monitoring your blood sugar? A case study of two ladies, A and B, may give you a glimpse into what you can expect. They both wore continuous glucose monitors for several days.

Charts show their hourly blood sugar readings at different times on the first day. The grey-shaded area defines the target range where most of the blood sugar readings should be.

- **Lady A, from midnight to 0800 hours**

Lady A's hourly blood sugar levels gradually dropped from midnight to 0400 hours as she slept. Her blood sugar started to rise about two hours before she woke up, indicating hormones signalled the liver to release stored sugar into the blood to prepare for the day.

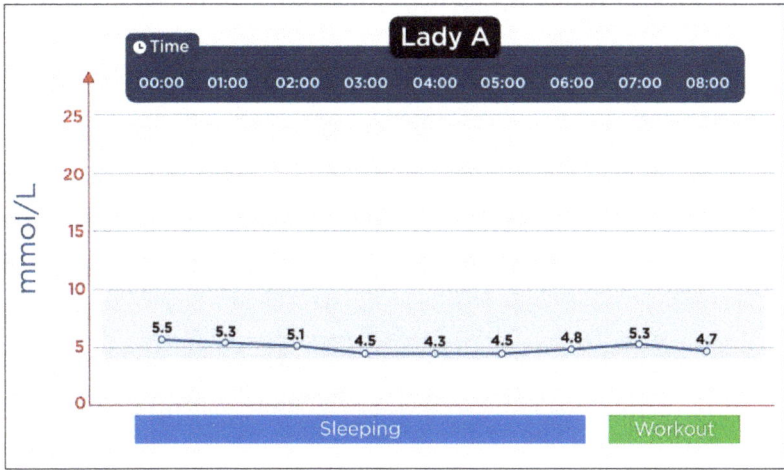

Her fasting blood sugar level when she woke up was in the normal range. A workout at 0630 hours induced the liver to release more sugar into the bloodstream, raising it to 5.3 mmol/L. Blood sugar levels steadily came down after the workout.

From midnight to 0800 hours, Lady A's blood sugar levels were in the target range.

- **Lady B, from midnight to 0800 hours**

Lady B's blood sugar levels tell a different story. Her blood sugar levels, whether asleep or awake, are above the target range, as indicated by the shaded area. Her fasting blood sugar level, 9.8 mmol/L at 0600 hours, is an indicator that her HbA1c is in the diabetic range.

Tea with two teaspoons of sugar shot her blood sugar to 11.9 mmol/l.

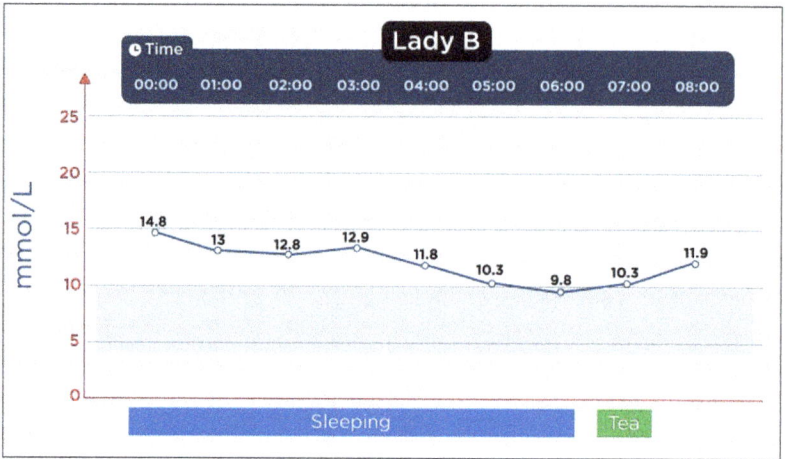

Lady B — Time 00:00 01:00 02:00 03:00 04:00 05:00 06:00 07:00 08:00. Values: 14.8, 13, 12.8, 12.9, 11.8, 10.3, 9.8, 10.3, 11.9 mmol/L. Sleeping / Tea.

- **Lady A, from 0800 to 1600 hours**

A bowl of porridge and black tea with no sugar raised Lady A's blood sugar levels to a peak of 7.4 mmol/L. Her blood sugar steadily came down to just above 4.0 mmol/L two hours after eating.

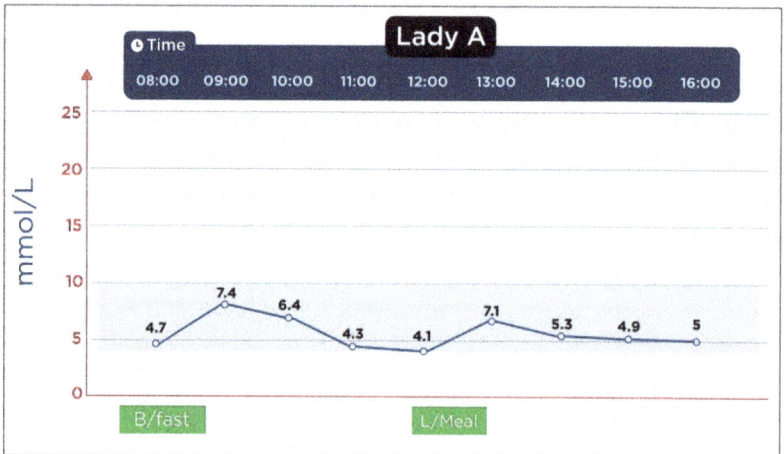

Lady A — Time 08:00 09:00 10:00 11:00 12:00 13:00 14:00 15:00 16:00. Values: 4.7, 7.4, 6.4, 4.3, 4.1, 7.1, 5.3, 4.9, 5 mmol/L. B/fast / L/Meal.

She had stir-fried green vegetables, two boiled eggs, and a mixture of sweet potato and yam at 1200. As expected, it raised her blood sugar. Her body gradually brought down the blood sugar level from 7.1 mmol/L to 4.9 mmol/L within two hours.

- **Lady B, from 0800 to 1600 hours**

Lady B's blood sugar levels remained above the normal range all morning. She had a brunch of toast with cheese, scrambled eggs, baked beans, and tea with two teaspoons of sugar after 1100 hours. Her blood sugar shot up to above 21 mmol/L.

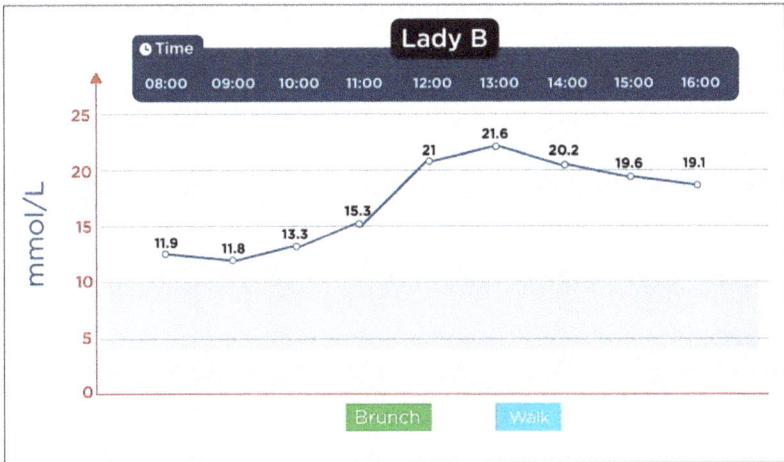

A 30-minute walk slightly reduced the blood sugar to 20.2 mmol/L. Her blood sugar remained above 19 mmol/L hours after eating and taking a walk.

- **Lady A, from 1600 to midnight**

At 1800 hours, Lady A had dinner consisting of stir-fried aboveground vegetables, roast chicken, half an avocado, a steamed piece of green banana, and half a plantain. The meal raised her blood sugar to 7.8 mmol/L.

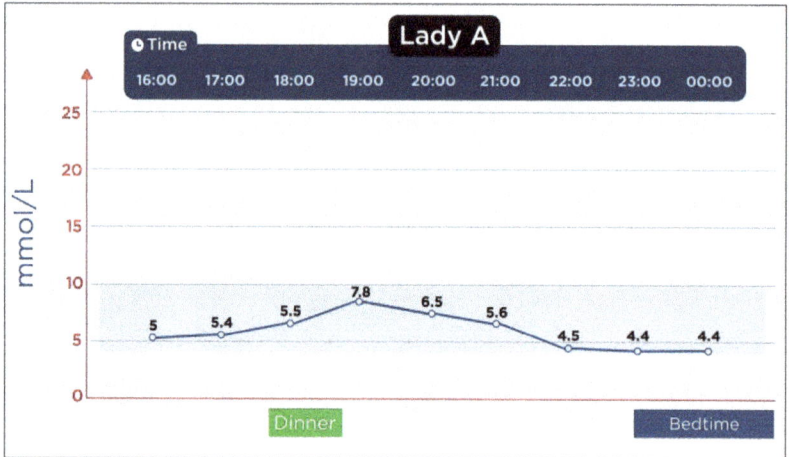

Once again, her blood sugar steadily came down after the meal and was 4.4 when she went to bed.

- **Lady B, from 1600 to midnight**

Lady B had chicken and mushroom stew and brown rice for dinner just before 1700 hours. The meal made her blood sugar shoot up to above 21 mmol/L, where it remained even two hours later.

Her blood sugar levels sharply fell before rising again to a concentration of 18.1 mmol/L when she went to bed.

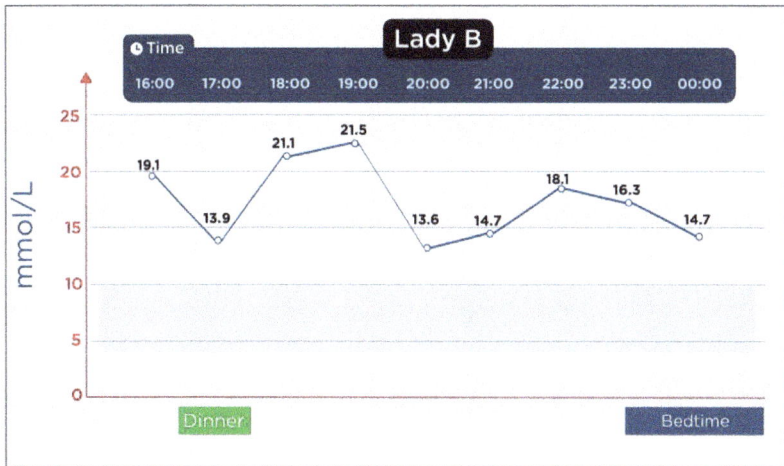

Insights gained

Lady A and Lady B accumulated invaluable information from their continuous glucose monitors on the first day. They learned how well their blood sugar was controlled and found out some of the factors that contributed to the fluctuations.

Self-awareness was the primary takeaway and provided pointers for what needed to be done next. Lady B immediately contacted her healthcare provider, and Lady A purposed to find out what she needed to continue doing and what to avoid.

Both ladies became drivers of their healthcare and partners to their healthcare providers.

Summary

Target blood sugar levels (Healthy Individual)

When	Measurement	
	mmol/L	mg/dL
Before meals	4.0 to 5.4	72 to 99
2 hours after meals	up to 7.8	up to 140

Target blood sugar levels (Type 2 Diabetes)

When	Measurement	
	mmol/L	mg/dL
Before meals	4.0 to 7.0 *	72 to 126 *
2 hours after meals	under 8.5 *	under 153 *
* Your healthcare provider may give you an individualised target after considering your age and any other illnesses or conditions you may have.		

Key Points

Testing your blood sugar levels opens a window through which you can see the inner workings of your blood sugar regulation. You no longer need to wait until you visit your healthcare provider to know how you are doing.

What story would your blood sugar readings tell? What story would you like them to tell?

CHAPTER 13

Managing High and Low Blood Sugar Levels

B lood sugar levels are rarely constant, as discussed in the last chapter. Both internal and external factors may cause either extreme.

Too much sugar in the bloodstream is called hyperglycaemia (hyper), and too little is called hypoglycaemia (hypo). You need to know the signals and stay prepared to manage both extremes if you have diabetes to prevent the development of diabetic emergencies.

High blood sugar (hyperglycaemia)

If you have type 2 diabetes, hyperglycaemia is a blood sugar reading of more than 7 mmol/L (126 mg/dL) before a meal or above 8.5 mmol/L (153 mg/dL) two hours after a meal.

And if you have pre-diabetes, a reading of more than 6 mmol/L (108 mg/dL) before a meal and more than 7.8 mmol/L (140 mg/dL) one hour after a meal is considered hyperglycaemia (NICE).

Some causes of high blood sugar

- Eating too much sugary or starchy food
- Stress
- Infections and being unwell
- Being less active than usual
- Missing doses of your diabetes medicine

Symptoms of high blood sugar

- Feeling very thirsty
- Peeing a lot
- Feeling weak or tired
- Blurred vision

Steps you can take to prevent high blood sugar

- Test your blood sugar regularly before and two hours after a meal.
- Take any diabetes medicines as prescribed.
- Avoid eating too much sugary or starchy food.
- Keep a food diary of everything you eat for a few days then reflect on which foods may be raising your blood sugar.
- Get adequate rest and sleep.
- Follow advice from your healthcare provider about what to do when you're ill.

Treating high blood sugar (hyper)

- Take diabetes medicines as prescribed.
- Follow sick-day rules given by your healthcare provider.
- Engage in physical activity, like walking, running, a workout, etc.
- If your blood sugar remains high, contact your healthcare provider.

***

Low blood sugar (hypoglycaemia)

A blood sugar level of less than 4 mmol/L (72 mg/dL) is low.

Symptoms of low blood sugar can be broken into two main groups, namely, early warning signs and late-onset signs.

You may experience some of these early warning signs:

- Increased hunger
- Difficulty concentrating
- Blurred vision
- Feeling shaky or trembling
- A fast or pounding heartbeat
- Getting easily irritated

If these early warning signs are not dealt with, you may go on to experience the following signs and symptoms:

- Feeling sleepy
- Being confused
- Looking like you are drunk
- Dizziness
- Seizures or fits
- Collapsing or passing out

Some causes of low blood sugar

- Too much diabetes medicine
- Taking diabetes medicines on an empty stomach
- Not eating enough or eating late
- Physical activity—a workout, gardening, etc.
- Drinking alcohol on an empty stomach

Steps you can take to prevent low blood sugar

- Eat your meals around the same time every day.
- Try to eat a similar amount at each meal.
- Check your blood sugar levels as recommended by your healthcare provider.
- Learn how to adjust your medicines if you are going to exercise.
- Consult your healthcare provider if you want to reduce your carbohydrate intake or plan to fast.
- Don't drink alcohol on an empty stomach.
- Contact your healthcare provider if you still experience hypos despite taking the above measures.

Treating a low blood sugar (hypo)

Take the following three steps:

Step 1: Take any one of the following fast-acting glucose sources (15 g).

- 1 mini can of Coke or half a can of full-sugar Coke/Sprite. (Do not use Coke Zero or Sprite Zero)
- 240 ml Lucozade
- A glass of fruit juice (apple or orange)
- 5 glucose or dextrose tablets
- 1 to 2 tubes of glucose gel
- 2 tablespoons of raisins

Resist the urge to eat or take more than the specified 15 g above. It may raise your blood sugar too high.

Step 2: Test your blood sugar after 15 minutes.

If it is still below 4 mmol/L (72 mg/dL), repeat step 1; otherwise, proceed to the next step.

Step 3: After a hypo

- If the hypo happens before a meal, have your meal.

- If the hypo happens in between meals, have a snack, e.g., tea with two crackers or biscuits, one-half of a sandwich, or two crackers with cheese. This should stop the blood sugar from going down again until you have your next meal.

***

Low blood sugar symptoms when blood sugar is more than 4 mmol/L

If your blood sugar is always high, then your body may feel like it is going into a hypo when the blood sugar level drops. Treat this as you would a hypo and consult your healthcare provider.

Low blood sugar unawareness

If you frequently get hypos, you may end up with what is called "hypoglycaemia unawareness." You may have no warning signs your blood sugar has dropped below 4 mmol/L. This can be dangerous as it can lead to severe hypoglycaemia. If left untreated, it can result in a diabetic coma. Consult your healthcare provider if your blood sugars are often low.

Diabetic emergencies

Untreated blood sugar extremes can lead to one of the following life-threatening emergencies:

- **Ketoacidosis**

Insufficient insulin may trigger the body to break down fat so fast it makes the blood acidic.
Urgent hospital treatment is required.

- **Hyperosmolar hyperglycaemic state (HHS)**

Blood sugar levels of more than 33 mmol/L (600 mg/dL) in a person with type 2 diabetes may lead to a hyperosmolar hyperglycaemic state (HHS). Symptoms include dehydration, vision problems, weakness, and an altered level of consciousness. Complications include seizures.
Urgent hospital treatment is required.

- **Severe hypoglycaemia**

A severe hypo is a low blood sugar that you cannot treat yourself. You may not be able to safely eat or drink.
Immediate medical care is required.
Your healthcare provider can issue you with a glucagon kit to be used by your family, friends, or carer in an emergency. They must know where to find the kit and how to use it.

Summary

Low blood sugar level (Hypo)

Type of Diabetes	Measurement	
	mmol/L	mg/dL
Any	Less than 4.0	Less than 72

High blood sugar levels (Prediabetes)

When	Measurement	
	mmol/L	mg/dL
Before food	Above 6.0	Above 108
1 hour after food	Above 7.8	Above 140

High blood sugar levels (Gestational Diabetes)

When	Measurement	
	mmol/L	mg/dL
Before food	Above 6.0	Above 108
1 hour after food	Above 7.8	Above 140

High blood sugar levels (Type 2 Diabetes)

When	Measurement	
	mmol/L	mg/dL
Before food	Above 7.0	Above 126
2 hours after food	Above 8.5	Above 153

Key Points

Managing high and low blood sugar levels is an essential part of self-care. Both extremes require a prompt informed response to prevent a diabetic emergency.

CHAPTER 14

Diabetes Medicines

Diabetes medicine prescriptions and treatment plans are tailored to meet the unique needs of each patient. Your healthcare provider considers your age, kidney function, blood test results, social circumstances, and other factors. So, the little tablet your friend or family member has been singing praises about may not be suitable for you.

Every diabetes medicine has an approved generic name. Different manufacturers may give it a different brand (trade) name. Generic names are used in this chapter to minimise confusion.

Though it is possible for some people to reverse type 2 diabetes, none of the current medicines are a cure. This chapter walks you through diabetes medicines from the vantage point of what they are meant to do, i.e., reduce insulin resistance, stimulate the pancreas to produce more insulin, slow down digestion and reduce appetite, get rid of excess sugar in the urine, and move excess sugar from the bloodstream into the cells.

Reduce insulin resistance

Metformin, which is taken in tablets, aids blood sugar control in the following two ways:
- Helps the body to absorb more sugar from the blood.
- Reduces the amount of sugar released by the liver.

Side effects include stomach upsets, vomiting, and diarrhoea.

On the plus side, *Metformin* reduces the risk of complications, does not cause weight gain, and is unlikely to cause low blood sugar (hypo).

Stimulate the pancreas to release more insulin

The class of tablets that include *Gliclazide, Glimepiride, Glibenclamide,* and *Tolbutamide* stimulate the pancreas to release more insulin.

While this reduces the blood sugar level, it increases the risk of low blood sugar. So, you need to regularly test your blood sugar levels if you take these tablets.

Side effects include stomach upset, diarrhoea, constipation, and weight gain.

Slow down digestion and reduce appetite

Another strategy is to slow down digestion so that the sugar from food takes longer to get into the blood, lowers the blood sugar and leads to weight loss.

Either tablets (known as Gliptins) or injections (referred to as GLP-1) are used. Gliptins include *Alogliptin, Linagliptin, Vildagliptin, and Sitagliptin*. And GLP-1s include *Trulicity, Ozempic, Victoza*, and *Semaglutide. Tirzapetide* is a combination of GLP-1 and GIP.

Side effects include nausea, diarrhoea, and stomach pain.

Get rid of excess sugar via the urine

Gliflozins, a class of tablets that include *Empagliflozin*, *Canagliflozin*, and *Dapagliflozin* prevent the reabsorption of sugar by the kidneys and increase the amount of sugar passed out in the urine.
Side effects include thrush and diabetic ketoacidosis if taken when you are on a very low-calorie diet.

Move excess sugar from the bloodstream into the cells

Your healthcare provider may start you on *insulin* injections if your blood sugar remains high despite the measures mentioned above. The full range of *insulins* is beyond the scope of this book. Below are a few examples.

Mealtime insulins, including *Actrapid*, *Humalog*, *Fiasp*, and *Apidra*, last about five to eight hours in the body.

Mixed mealtime insulins, usually taken twice daily and lasting about 12 to 16 hours, include *Novomix 30* and *Humulin M3*.

Medium-to long-acting insulins like *Humulin I*, *Insulatard*, *Lantus*, *Tresiba*, and *Toujeo* taken once or twice a day last 12 to 36 hours.

Common side effects include weight gain and low blood sugar.

Myths about diabetes medicines

Some diabetes patients will not take prescribed medicines because they sincerely believe that they won't be able to stop once they start taking them. Some think they are the cause of amputations, erectile dysfunction, and a significant number of patients have been led to believe that pharmaceutical companies are withholding the cure for diabetes to make money.

Takeaways

Diabetes medicines are useful in bringing blood sugar levels down and act on various parts of the body to achieve their intended purpose. They do need to be taken with caution and with adjustments to diet and lifestyle for them to work well.

Self-medicating can lead to unexpected complications. All medicines must be prescribed by qualified healthcare professionals.

CHAPTER 15

Herbs and Spices

This chapter discusses the use of herbs and spices to naturally lower and control blood sugar levels. Herbal therapies are not regulated in the same way as prescribed medications. It cannot be stressed enough that herbs and spices are not a substitute for the prescribed medicines listed in the last chapter.

It is important to speak to your pharmacist before taking them because they may affect the way your diabetes medicines work. Consider keeping a diary of how your body responds and discuss this with your pharmacist as needed.

Bitter melon

Bitter melon gets its name from its taste. It is commonly used as a vegetable in East Africa, Asia, the Caribbean, and South America.

Research has shown bitter melon has insulin-like properties that help manage blood sugar. It is taken in its natural form as a vegetable, in tablets, or as tea. There are no standard doses for medical treatment at this stage, and it must be taken with caution.

Side effects include diarrhoea, low blood sugar, and liver damage.

Cinnamon

Cinnamon is a sweet spice obtained from the inner bark of wild cinnamon trees that grow in South America, the Caribbean, and Asia. It is sold as cinnamon sticks, powder, tea, oil, and tablet supplements.

It is used in cooking and baking. Some clinical studies suggest cinnamon may help reduce blood sugar levels and increase insulin sensitivity.

Though cinnamon has additional health benefits, caution is advised before taking it with other herbs, spices, or diabetes medicines.

Aloe vera

Aloe vera is a juicy plant that is incorporated into a multitude of personal care products.

Research suggests that aloe vera juice can help improve blood sugar levels and the effects of the so-called diabetic foot. Aloe vera is consumed as a juice extracted from the plant, in powder form, or as capsule supplements.

Medical advice is recommended before taking it to make sure it won't conflict with any medicines you may already be taking.

Side effects include abdominal pain, diarrhoea, and low blood sugar.

Fenugreek seeds

The fenugreek plant is used in herbal medicine. The seeds and powder are also used in Asian dishes for their slightly sweet and nutty taste.

Fenugreek, which is high in insoluble fibre, slows down digestion and the absorption of sugar into the blood. This helps lower blood sugar. The seeds are also soaked in water and the juice is drunk either hot or cold.

Side effects include stomach pain, skin irritation, and diarrhoea.

Okra (lady fingers)

Okra is a plant with edible green-seed pods. It is cultivated in warm-to-hot regions around the world. Though it is a fruit, okra is eaten as a vegetable.

Okra's high fibre reduces the rate at which sugar is absorbed from the intestines and, therefore, lowers blood sugar levels. It can be added to soups, stews, or fried on its own. Alternatively, okra pieces can be added to water overnight and the juice consumed in the morning.

Though it is generally safe to eat, side effects in some people include gas, diarrhoea, and stomach cramps.

Moringa

Moringa is called a superfood for good reasons. The leaves contain more vitamin A than carrots, more vitamin C than oranges, more iron than spinach, more calcium than milk, and more potassium than bananas. It is widely cultivated across the tropics.

Studies show that the insulin-like properties found in moringa may help lower blood sugar. Leaves can be used to make tea or eaten as a vegetable. Fruit from the pods can also be eaten.

It is advisable to consult your pharmacist for the right dosage for you.

Summary

- There are many more herbs and spices that people use for good health and to manage diabetes.
- The side effects listed here are not conclusive. Some herbs and spices may interact with other medicines you may be taking for other conditions, and some are not suitable for pregnancy.

Herbs and spices are not a substitute for managing your diet and lifestyle. It is advisable to consult your pharmacist before you consider taking them.

CHAPTER 16

Low-carb Dieting and Fasting

Low-carb dieting and fasting are gaining popularity as effective ways to control blood sugar and weight. They both trigger the breakdown of stored fat to provide energy for the body.

Your options depend on your current state of health and the medicines you are taking. You may be required to eat regularly if you are on diabetes medication. It is, therefore, necessary to consult your healthcare provider if you are considering either dieting or fasting.

1. Low-carbohydrate diets

Studies have shown that low-carbohydrate diets are useful in managing weight and improving well-being. Some people have achieved remission from diabetes and stopped all medicines. We explore three main types of low-carbohydrate diets: total diet replacement, the ketogenic diet and conventional low-carbohydrate diet.

1.1 Total diet replacement (TDR), 800 calories/day

Total diet replacement, a very low-calorie diet, is usually done under the supervision of your healthcare provider.

In the first three months, one has low-starch vegetables and a liquid diet of soups and shakes three times a day. Diabetes and associated medicines, e.g., blood pressure or water tablets, may need to be stopped. Your healthcare team will provide guidance.

Solid food is slowly reintroduced into meals after three months.

Some of those undertaking this diet have lost up to 13 kg in three months and, in some cases, brought their diabetes into remission.

This diet is not for everyone. While some do very well, many drop out. Among those that last the distance, some have commented on how difficult it is to maintain the weight loss after the initial three-month period, so some have gone back to medicines and regained the weight. The good news is others have done well, kept the weight off, and are still in remission today.

1.2 Ketogenic diet

The "keto" diet, as it is popularly known, is a very low-carb and high-fat diet. It has many similarities to Atkins and other low-carb diets. It drastically cuts back on carbohydrate intake and replaces it with fat.

This causes your body to go into a metabolic state, called ketosis, in which it becomes more efficient at breaking down fat for energy.

This diet has been shown to significantly lower blood sugar and shift the body from using carbohydrates as its primary source of energy, thereby reducing the need for medicines.

1.3 Conventional Low-carbohydrate diet

A conventional low-carb diet gives prominence to low-starchy vegetables and foods high in protein and fats. There is no standard definition of this diet. Some researchers recommend up to 130 grams of carbohydrate per day. To put this into context, a slice of bread can contain up to 20 grams of carbohydrate. This diet is recommended by healthcare professionals for people with diabetes because it helps to reduce and maintain blood sugar levels, is sustainable, leads to weight loss and improves overall health and well-being.

2. Fasting

Fasting has been part of religious and spiritual practices for centuries on almost every continent.

Two ways of fasting are explored.

2.1 Intermittent fasting or time-restricted eating

Intermittent fasting entails eating during a specific period, followed by a set period of not eating. It has no restrictions on what to eat, only when you should eat. Common methods include alternate-day fasting (for 24 hours) and daily time-restricted fasting (e.g., 16-hour fasting and 8-hour eating).

2.2 The 5:2 Diet

This plan involves eating normally for 5 days of the week and fasting for 2. During the 2 days of fasting, you eat less. On fasting days, women typically consume 500 calories, while men consume 600 calories. The fasting days do not have to be one after another and can change from week to week to suit your lifestyle and circumstances.

Benefits of fasting

There is no cost to fasting. It reduces the body's resistance to insulin and promotes the breakdown of fat. Through a process called autophagy, the body gets rid of dead cells and promotes the regeneration of new cells.

Summary

Countless diets are promoted today. We have only scratched the surface. Furthermore, it's worth remembering that a diet is a set of rules that have been followed by many or a few to achieve an outcome like losing weight.

Find what works best for you, your lifestyle, and your family. You may find that you need a hybrid diet. For example, if you tend to snack, eating only at mealtimes may be the only change you need to make. Do your research and consult your healthcare team before you start.

CHAPTER 17

Making the Most of Your Healthcare Appointment

Have you ever left your healthcare appointment, thinking, "I wish I had asked this or that? How could I forget?" Join the club. A time-limited appointment often makes it difficult to ask all the questions you may have.

Preparation is key to making the most of your short appointment.

Be prepared

- Note down any questions you may have about your blood test results, symptoms, and concerns.
- Make a list of all your medicines (not just diabetes medications), including vitamins, minerals, or dietary supplements, if any.
- Record blood sugar readings in your diary or download and print out your most recent meter results.
- If you use a continuous glucose monitor, record as much information as you can on the app or on paper.

- Consider keeping a three-day food, activity, sleep, stress, or illness diary.
- Write down any specific symptoms that you have experienced, e.g., numbness, tingling in your feet, etc.
- Be ready with one or two main issues that you want to focus on and discuss during your visit.
- Consider inviting a family member or friend along to take notes, listen, and be supportive.

During the visit

- Ask your questions, verify your understanding, and write down the answers.
- Ask about treatment options and what you can do to get your blood sugar, blood pressure, and cholesterol into target.
- Find out and understand your lab and examination results.
- Be prepared to take off your shoes and socks to have your feet checked.
- Obtain reasons for a change of medicines, what they are meant to address, and known side effects.

After the visit

- Follow up with your healthcare provider for any laboratory test results or examinations that were done.
- Write down or download your results to help you keep track.
- Continue to monitor changes to your diet, lifestyle, or any side effects of new medicines.
- Call your healthcare provider if you have questions.

Summary

Your visit to your healthcare provider is an excellent opportunity to fill in any gaps you may have in your diabetes knowledge and to learn how you can be better equipped to manage your condition. It is also a good opportunity for your healthcare provider to learn how they can serve you better and address any issues or difficulties you may be going through. Preparation is key.

CHAPTER 18

Safe Driving

Having diabetes does not mean you should give up driving. However, it does add a layer of responsibility to ensure your safety and that of other road users.

Drivers on insulin and other diabetes medicines have a risk of low blood sugar (hypoglycaemia). The most significant driving hazard is unrecognised hypoglycaemia, which affects your ability to decide when it is safe to drive.

The risk is higher for commercial vehicle drivers because the consequences of an accident are likely to be more serious.

Licensing rules for people with diabetes vary from country to country and, sometimes, state to state. It is important to find out the rules and regulations applicable where you are.

Your responsibilities

- Understand rules and regulations as they apply in your country or state. In most countries, it is your responsibility to inform the Driver and Vehicle Licensing

Agency if you are on medicines that can cause hypoglycaemia.

- Inform your motor vehicle insurer about your diabetes to avoid problems with insurance claims.
- Have regular medical diabetes reviews.
- Actively manage your blood sugar levels.
- Report incidents of hypoglycaemia to your healthcare provider.
- Take your medicines as prescribed.
- Undergo a medical examination as often as is required in your country to assess fitness to drive.

Before driving

- Ensure you have fast-acting carbohydrates like glucose tablets, a juice box, and extra snacks in the car.
- Have a spare blood sugar monitor or meter and extra test strips in the car.
- Wear your diabetes medical identification if you have one.
- Ensure you have a planned meal before setting off.
- Check your blood sugar.

When not to drive

- Your blood sugar is below 5 mmol/L (90 mg/dL).
- Your meal is delayed.
- You feel unwell.
- You feel numbness or weakness in your limbs.

Checks on the road

- Stop to check your blood sugar regularly if you are driving for a prolonged period.

- Do not get back on the road if your blood sugar is less than 5 mmol/L (90 mg/dL).

If you have a hypo

1. Pull over as soon as it is safe to do so.
2. Switch off the ignition and remove the key to show you are not in charge of the car.
3. Get into the passenger seat.
4. Treat the hypo as advised.
5. Wait until the blood sugar level is above 6 mmol/L (108 mg/dL) and do not drive for at least 45 minutes to give the brain ample time to recover.

Staying safe on the road

- Always keep hypo treatments in the car.
- Do not drive if your blood sugar is less than 5.0 mmol/L (90 mg/dL).
- If your reading is between 4.0 and 5.0 mmol/L (72 and 90 mg/dL), eat a small starchy snack like half a sandwich with protein.
- If your blood sugar is less than 4 mmol/L (72 mg/dL), treat the hypo and do not drive for at least 45 minutes after you have recovered.

CHAPTER 19

Travelling Tips

Having diabetes should not hinder you from travelling to any destination in the world. With careful planning, you can manage diabetes anywhere just as well as you can at home.

Though not everyone follows the traditional travel wisdom of "Take half as many clothes and twice as much money as you think you'll need for any holiday," nothing can be left to chance if you are on diabetes medicines.

You are urged to carefully plan and prepare for your holiday once you know where you are going, how you're travelling, and how long you will be away.

Four weeks before travelling . . .

- Research diabetes services available where you are going. Your healthcare provider may be able to give you some pointers. The national diabetes association in the country you are visiting can give you useful contact details.
- See your healthcare provider for a general health check and ensure your diabetes is under control.

- Request a travel letter that states you have diabetes, any other conditions you may have, and the medications you are taking. Ask your healthcare provider to use the generic names of medicines because brand names can vary from country to country. The letter will be useful if you need emergency care.
- Get prescriptions for medicines you use and at least twice as much diabetes medications as you think you will need. The place you're visiting may not have the supplies.
- Ask your doctor for medications to prevent motion sickness and diarrhoea.
- Make sure you have some type of medical identification to wear or carry with you that states you have diabetes. This can be a bracelet or necklace or a card that you carry in your wallet. Ensure your name, address, phone number, and your healthcare provider's name and phone number are on the card. Write the kind and amount of diabetes and other medicines you take.
- Ensure you get the immunisations advised for your destination and plan to take the records with you.
- Make an appointment with your dietician and diabetes nurse to discuss when and what to eat if you are travelling across time zones and when to take insulin and medicines.
- If you are travelling by air, find out if the airline serves meals, the times they are served, and the meal options.
- Check current regulations about carry-on bags with your airline or the Transportation Security Administration.

Your carry-on bag

The carry-on bag will have your diabetes medicines, including pills, insulin, and any other injectables you will need for your trip. It is not for checking in on a plane, train, or bus. Important reminders include the following:

- The travel letter from your doctor authorising you to carry medicines on you through airport and train station security.
- You need a special insulated travel pack to keep insulin and other injectables between 2°C and 8°C (36°F and 46°F).
- Pack a glucagon kit if you are at risk for low blood glucose.
- Pack an extra meter and batteries, extra test strips, and extra lancets.
- If you use a continuous glucose monitor, ensure you carry extra glucose sensors.
- Pack ketone strips if you take insulin or medicines that can increase the risk of diabetic ketoacidosis.
- Pack pump supplies if you use an insulin pump.
- Pack snacks that contain carbohydrates, such as granola bars or dried fruit, in case of meal delays or low blood sugar.

On the way . . .

- Have your medical identification card that specifies your condition on you and wear a bracelet or necklace with the same facts.
- Do not skip meals or snacks.
- Remember to check your blood glucose levels every three to six hours.

- Wear comfortable shoes and socks and check your feet frequently for blisters. Get treatment if even minor foot problems develop.
- Tell people you travel with that you have diabetes. Explain how to recognise low blood sugar and how to treat it.
- Do your best to follow your meal and physical activity plan as closely as possible.

At your destination

- Regularly check your blood sugar and follow your healthcare provider's instructions to treat highs or lows.
- Avoid overeating. Stick to healthier choices or a low-carb menu.
- Avoid exposure to high temperatures. It may change how your body uses insulin.
- Find out the locations of the nearest pharmacy and general practitioner.
- Learn useful phrases in the local language.

When you return . . .

- If you have been away for several months, visit your healthcare provider for an up-to-date checkup and blood test.
- If you are on insulin and have been to a hot climate, you may need to increase your doses.
- Check your blood sugar levels more frequently as you adjust to your diet and lifestyle.

Unplanned travel

If you are likely to travel in an emergency, it is advisable to stay ready by keeping a carry-on bag stocked with essential items.

Takeaways

Travelling when you have diabetes needs some planning before you leave to allow you the freedom to enjoy your time away. Being prepared means that even if you are taken ill while you are away, you have the contacts and medicines you need.

CHAPTER 20

The Annual Review

An annual review is a must-have if you have diabetes, are in remission, have had pre-diabetes, or have had a past diagnosis of gestational diabetes (diabetes in pregnancy).

Unlike other visits to your healthcare provider, the focus of the annual review is proactive care. The priority is to identify and prevent health problems before they become critical.

Hence, regular periodic tests and assessments throughout the year help to paint a complete picture of your journey and guide the way forward.

The type of annual review you have depends on your health status.

Type 2 diabetes (including remission) annual review

If you are in remission, a review is still advised. A typical review can be made up of the following:

a) Review of test results and examination

Feedback is given on the following test results:

- **Average blood sugar (HbA1c)**

  Your current HbA1c is reviewed, and previous test results are analysed to find a trend. The most recent blood sugar monitor (or continuous glucose monitor) readings and notes are also evaluated using your observations of the effects of food, medicines, stress, and any other factors.

- **Blood pressure (BP)**

  The latest blood pressure taken in the clinic is reviewed and compared with any previous results. You may also be asked to provide home blood pressure readings, current and previous, especially if you suffer from white coat syndrome (anxiety in the clinic inflates blood pressure readings).

- **Blood fats (cholesterol)**

  Current and previous blood fat results are assessed in the context of your diet.

- **Kidney function (eGfr) and urine protein level (ACR)**

  Kidney function test results from urine and blood samples are assessed in relation to previous tests if any.

- **Body fat (BMI and waist circumference)**

  Your current body mass index (BMI) and waist circumference are assessed and contrasted with previous readings if any.

- **Eye screening**

  Your eye screening results are considered in the context of your latest HbA1c and blood pressure.

- **Feet and legs check (skin, circulation, and nerves)**

  Be ready to take off your shoes and socks. Your feet are checked for wounds, broken skin, and signs of circulation problems and nerve damage.

- **Injection sites (if you are on injectable diabetes medicines).**

  Injection sites are examined to ensure the risk of lumps is minimal.

b) Medicines assessment

- **Review of diabetes and related medicines**

  Diabetes, blood pressure, and cholesterol medicines and doses are reviewed, and their effectiveness is assessed.

- **Management of low blood sugar (hypos), if any**

  The frequency and times of hypos are assessed in relation to your diabetes medicine doses, mealtimes, and other factors.

c) Diabetes education needs

Diabetes knowledge gaps are assessed, and education needs are identified.

d) Your input

Your input may include the following:

- Your general well-being and how you are managing
- Physical activity regime and challenges if any
- Your general diet in relation to your blood sugar control
- Your smoking status
- Alcohol consumption and its effects on blood sugars
- Sexual health issues, including erectile dysfunction (for men) and plans to conceive (for women)
- Dental checkups and issues, if any
- Mental health issues, including diabetes distress, depression, unmanaged stress, bereavement, etc.

e) Goal setting and care planning

Your priorities and the lane you choose for remission or management, drive the most important part of the annual review—looking ahead.

You and your healthcare provider agree to set measurable goals for the year, which may include your target HbA1c, blood pressure, cholesterol, and body mass index (BMI).

An action plan that includes personalised care may include some of the following:

- Adjustments to current medicines
- Increase in physical activities
- Changes to diet
- Referrals to other specialists as required, such as nephrologist (kidney), endocrinologist (diabetes specialist), diabetes consultant nurse, psychologist or mental health nurse, podiatrist (foot care specialist)
- Structured diabetes education courses

Review dates are agreed upon and set.

Annual review for pre-diabetes and diabetes in pregnancy

A past diagnosis of either pre-diabetes or gestational diabetes (diabetes in pregnancy) necessitates an annual review because of the high risk of developing type 2 diabetes. The primary focus of the review is your lifestyle. A typical review is comprised of the following:

a) Assessment of test results

The latest test results should ideally show you are moving away from the high-risk lane. Where you are is indicated by the following test results

- Your current average blood sugar (HbA1c) is assessed and contrasted to previous tests, if any.
- Your blood pressure now and previous readings, if any, are reviewed in relation to your HBA1c.
- Your blood fat (cholesterol) test results are assessed and contrasted to your HBA1c and previous readings, if any.
- Body fat indicated by your current body mass index (BMI) and waist circumference is assessed and contrasted with previous readings, if any.

b) Your input

The more essential information you give your healthcare provider, the more comprehensive the guidance. Your input may include the following:

- Your general well-being
- Physical activities schedule and challenges, if any
- Your general diet and appreciation of portion sizes to control blood sugars
- Your smoking status

- Alcohol consumption and effects on blood sugars
- Plans to conceive (if you are a woman of childbearing age)

c) Goal setting and care planning

Your priorities and choice of lane, preventive or pre-diabetes, drive your target goals and care plan for the year ahead. Measurable goals for the year may include targets for HbA1c, blood pressure, cholesterol, and body mass index (BMI).

The action plan for the year may include the following:

- Medication prescriptions
- Physical activity recommendations
- Changes to diet
- Referrals to other specialists as required, such as nephrologist (kidney), clinical psychologist, mental health nurse, dietician/nutrition adviser, and hypertension clinic
- Structured diabetes prevention education courses

Takeaways

- An annual review is essential if you have type 2 diabetes, are in remission, have had pre-diabetes, or have had a past diagnosis of gestational diabetes.
- The focus of the annual review is proactive care.
- You and your healthcare provider jointly contribute to the annual review. Your preparation is key to its effectiveness.

CHAPTER 21

Managing Type 2 Diabetes in Older Adults

Data in the public domain indicates that type 2 diabetes is on the rise among senior citizens worldwide. The percentage is judged to be higher among individuals of African, Middle Eastern, and South Asian descent. It is so prevalent in some communities that it gives the impression that diabetes is synonymous with aging. Poor healthcare services and healthcare inequalities in some regions raise the risk of complications and diabetes-related deaths.

Reasons for the rise in senior citizens

Reasons for the increase in type 2 diabetes in senior citizens include the following:

- Tendency to get less active as one gets older. Some health conditions, like arthritis, limit mobility.
- Decreased or poor-quality sleep. It hampers blood sugar control and increases the risk of insulin resistance.

- Health conditions like high blood pressure, high cholesterol, and kidney disease hinder blood sugar control.

Extended family support

Most senior citizens with diabetes and other ailments are traditionally cared for at home, in line with the extended family cultures of Africa, the Middle East, and South Asia. It is just as well because some older adults find it challenging to take daily medicines and regularly monitor blood sugars.

The quality of home care is variable. Challenges include inadequate knowledge of diabetes management, limited access to blood sugar monitors or continuous glucose monitors (CGM), and resistance to change. Despite best intentions, the wider family does not always know how best to be supportive of an "aging elder."

Top tips include the following:

- **Healthcare appointments**

  Keeping appointments is an important part of diabetes management. Helping a loved one prepare questions ahead of time, accompanying the older adult to appointments, and taking notes on the day provide moral support and present opportunities to learn more about the condition.

- **Medication**

  Help ensure that medications are taken at the right time in the correct doses.

- **Food**

  Follow the healthcare provider's eating plans and recommendations. It would be helpful if the whole family made changes to their lifetime eating patterns.
  Pay attention to portion sizes and the timing of meals.

- **Increasing activity**

  Assist the senior citizen to follow the prescribed activity programme. Going out for a walk with a loved one is mutually beneficial.

- **Feet inspection**

  Routinely inspect your loved one's feet.

Self-care

Whether or not you have the extended family's support, it is important that you assume as much responsibility as you can. Be knowledgeable about what you need to do to live a healthy life with diabetes. What you need to keep an eye on includes the following:

- **Average blood sugar (HBA1c)**

  The efforts you make to manage your condition are reflected in your average blood sugar (HbA1c) over the last two to three months. Having it checked every three to six months enables you to set your bearings.
  Your healthcare provider will set a unique HBA1c target considering your age and other conditions you may have.

- **Blood sugar levels**

  Be familiar with your blood sugar targets. Monitor your blood sugar levels as advised by your healthcare provider. If you are using a blood glucose meter, make sure it is working well.

  On the average, your blood sugar targets will be in this range:

  - between 4.0 and 7.2 mmol/L (72 and 130 mg/dL) before meals and
  - less than 10 mmol/L (180 mg/dL) two hours after eating.

  Your healthcare provider may give you an individualised target after considering your age and any other illnesses or conditions you may have.

  Contact your healthcare provider if your readings are above target.

- **Medication**

  Taking your medicines is a must. Make an appointment to see your healthcare provider if taking them starts to feel like a chore, you are finding it difficult to swallow, there are so many tablets it is a challenge to keep track, or you are experiencing other difficulties. Your medicines for diabetes and other conditions may be adjusted to make life easier for you. A combination of reminder alarms, calendar notes, and a pill box organiser can help you keep track of your medicines.

- **Nutrition**

  Ensure you have balanced and nutritious meals. Use the plate method to control portions, especially carbohydrates.

  Consult your healthcare provider for a referral to a dietitian if you need help to select the right foods. Make an appointment with your dentist if oral health issues are making it difficult for you to eat.

  Avoid skipping meals. It puts you at risk of low blood sugar.

- **Physical activity**

  Staying active is essential as you get older. Arthritis, osteoporosis, joint problems, back pain, and other ailments may make it difficult to remain active. Do as much as your health issues allow.

  Your options include walking, gardening, yoga, swimming, cycling, and going up and down the stairs at home. Remember to keep an eye on your blood sugar.

- **Low blood sugar**

  Low blood sugar (hypo) is one of the side effects of diabetes medicines. Some health conditions (e.g., kidney disease) can raise the risk of low blood sugar.

  You must check your blood sugar before and after physical activities. If you have had a hypo, contact your healthcare provider.

- **Foot care**

  Check your feet regularly and raise the alarm if you have any wounds or blisters. Wear loose-fitting shoes and slippers in the house or outside.

Summary

Target blood sugar levels

When	Measurement	
	mmol/L	mg/dL
Before meals	4.0 to 7.2 *	72 to 130 *
2 hours after meals	less than 10 *	less than 180 *
Your healthcare provider may give you an individualised target after considering your age and any other illnesses or conditions you may have.		

Key Points

- Keep appointments with your healthcare providers.
- Be mindful of the individualised blood sugar targets set for you.
- Contact your healthcare provider if you experience low blood sugar.
- Eat regularly and do not skip meals.
- Stay as active as your health issues allow.
- Check your feet regularly.

CHAPTER 22

Making Lasting Changes

The fight for good health and a quality life extends beyond type 2 diabetes. However, the primary battlefield is the mind. For example, the food on your dinner plate is the result of a series of subconscious decisions that influence the grocery list, the size of pots, the quantities cooked, and how much is dished out. Understanding this combat zone puts you in a better position to make informed choices for yourself and your loved ones.

The battleground

- Need to instill the notion that type 2 diabetes is preventable, reversible, and stoppable in its tracks. Everyone has a role to play in debunking the view that type 2 diabetes is inevitable.
- Accept it is time we reviewed our eating habits and our favourite staple foods may not be as good as perceived. The more carbohydrates we eat, the more we put a strain on the internal system that regulates blood sugar, and the more we put vital organs at risk.
- Be on guard against the pitfalls and health risks associated with survival mode. It is advisable to explore the reasons behind established practices.

- Understand the health risks associated with excess weight. Help influence what a "good body" looks like.
- Probe cultural and religious beliefs that blame all illnesses, including type 2 diabetes, on mystical enemies.

Make your health a top priority

If there is only one thing you can take away from this book, let it be the need to assume responsibility for your own healthcare. You are the only one who can make your health the top priority. Healthcare professionals, family, and hired help cannot put you first.

You only have one body, one set of organs, and one shot at life. Your life's goals are dependent on your well-being. How you look after yourself today determines your tomorrow, whatever your current state of health.

Make it a lifetime commitment to treat yourself like someone you love. Purpose to take better care of your health and be kinder to your own body. Remember, self-care is a lifetime journey.

Your journey

Managing your health and diabetes is a balancing act. The diabetes navigation wheel below has five key areas: eat well, stay active, recharge regularly, keep up-to-date, and stay connected to help you maintain your balance.

It is helpful to remember that you did not get where you are overnight. Do what you can sustain and build on.

Gently steer in the direction the situation demands. Make changes in small steps.

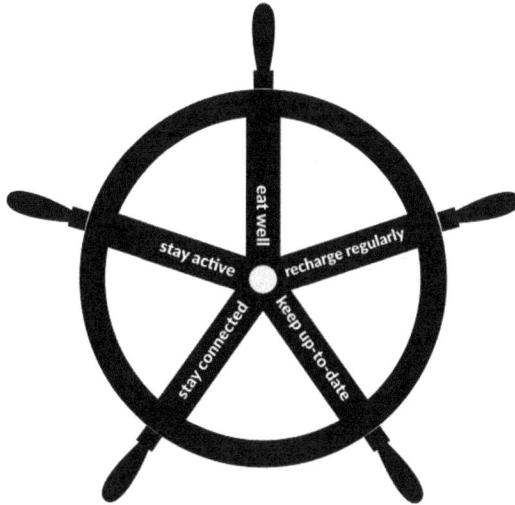

The most important thing is that you remain on the road.

Eat well

Be well-informed about foods that are good for you, the recommended quantities, and what to minimise. The following are key points to remember:
- Eat foods as close to their natural state as possible.
- Follow the plate method when planning your meals.

Stay active

Incorporate physical activity into every aspect of your life. If you don't stay physically active, you may lose your ability to do so.

Recharge regularly

Make rest, relaxation, and sleep an integral part of your self-care by scheduling time to engage in activities you enjoy and practising good sleep hygiene to ensure you get adequate rest.

Stay connected

While staying connected includes family, friends, colleagues, and so on, the biggest connection you can make is with yourself.

- Take time out for yourself to listen to your body, be on the lookout for your mental well-being and seek help as soon as you realise there is a problem.
- Get to know the type of person you are and focus on your strengths and weaknesses to achieve your goals.
- Monitor your health and progress by making the most of the healthcare technology available.
- Join groups and communities of like-minded people.
- Attend all your appointments with your healthcare provider.

Keep up-to-date

Millions are invested in diabetes research worldwide. Information and knowledge are constantly evolving.

- Carefully choose your sources of the latest diabetes information.
- Plug into the latest at your national diabetes association and healthcare providers.
- Become a diabetes advocate by sharing the knowledge you have gained. For example, if you found the tips and strategies laid out in this book useful, consider recommending or gifting a copy to 6 people you care about and want greater health and wellbeing for. They could be family, friends, neighbours, or colleagues. Someone's health and life may be forever changed for the better.

Write down names of up to 6 people you will recommend or give a copy of this book to:

1._____

2._____

3._____

4._____

5._____

6._____

Thank you for your valuable time. I look forward to reading your improved health story!

To YOUR health and well-being

Tembi Chinaire

Index

Acknowledgments

Thank you

Deep gratitude to colleagues and friends on the frontline of the war against type 2 diabetes from whom I learn daily.

Special thanks to the beta readers who read draft chapters and offered valuable feedback: Dr Paula Fernandes, Dr Nooses Hirani, Chakshu Sharma, Sibongile Thembi Xaba, Dr Chad Hockey and Dr Adel Isaak.

To my amazing husband and friend, Chris, thank you for your support and bringing out the best in me. And to my wonderful son, Ruvheneko, thank you for cheering me on from the sidelines and giving me much needed boost of energy.

Data Sources

Diabetes UK, National Institute for Health and Care Excellence (NICE) diabetes guidelines, American Diabetes Association, International Diabetes Federation (IDF), and World Health Organisation (WHO) provided useful reference materials.

Teaspoons of sugar reference values for foods were taken using an average of commercially available products or calculated from recipes and food labels. Some values have been estimated using similar products. Please note that the values in this book are to be used as a guide only.

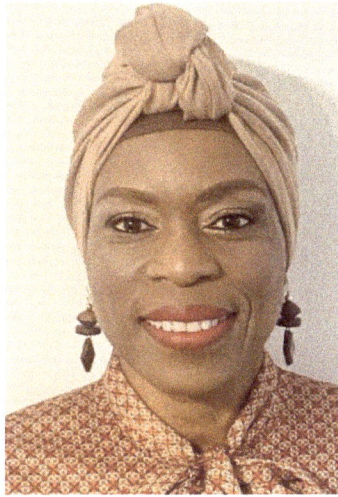

ABOUT THE AUTHOR

TEMBI CHINAIRE is a diabetes educator, certified nutrition adviser and diabetes consultant nurse. She has extensive public and private healthcare experience, having set up or led diabetes services for over 14 years in England, UK.

Tembi has written and delivered tailored diabetes education programmes in the Middle East, Africa, and the UK.

She is committed to equipping people with the tools to become drivers of their own healthcare so they can live richer and more fulfilling lives.

Tembi is passionate about preventing type 2 diabetes and reducing the onset and progression of complications for those already diagnosed with the disease.

She is a Florence Nightingale Travel Scholarship winner and is a current member of the National Institute for Health and Care Excellence (NICE) Diabetes Guidelines Update Committee in England, UK.

www.ingramcontent.com/pod-product-compliance
Lightning Source LLC
Chambersburg PA
CBHW051246020426

42333CB00025B/3079